INTERMITTENT FASTING FOR WOMEN OVER 50

How to Weight Loss and

Burn Fat After Menopause

with a 5-Step Metabolism

Scientific Method and

Slowing Down Aging

with Easy Strategies

Jennifer Campbell

The information herein is offered for informational purposes solely, and is universal as so. The presentation of the information is without contract or any type of guarantee assurance.

The trademarks that are used are without any consent, and the publication of the trademark is without permission or backing by the trademark owner. All trademarks and brands within this book are for clarifying purposes only and are the owned by the owners themselves, not affiliated with this document.

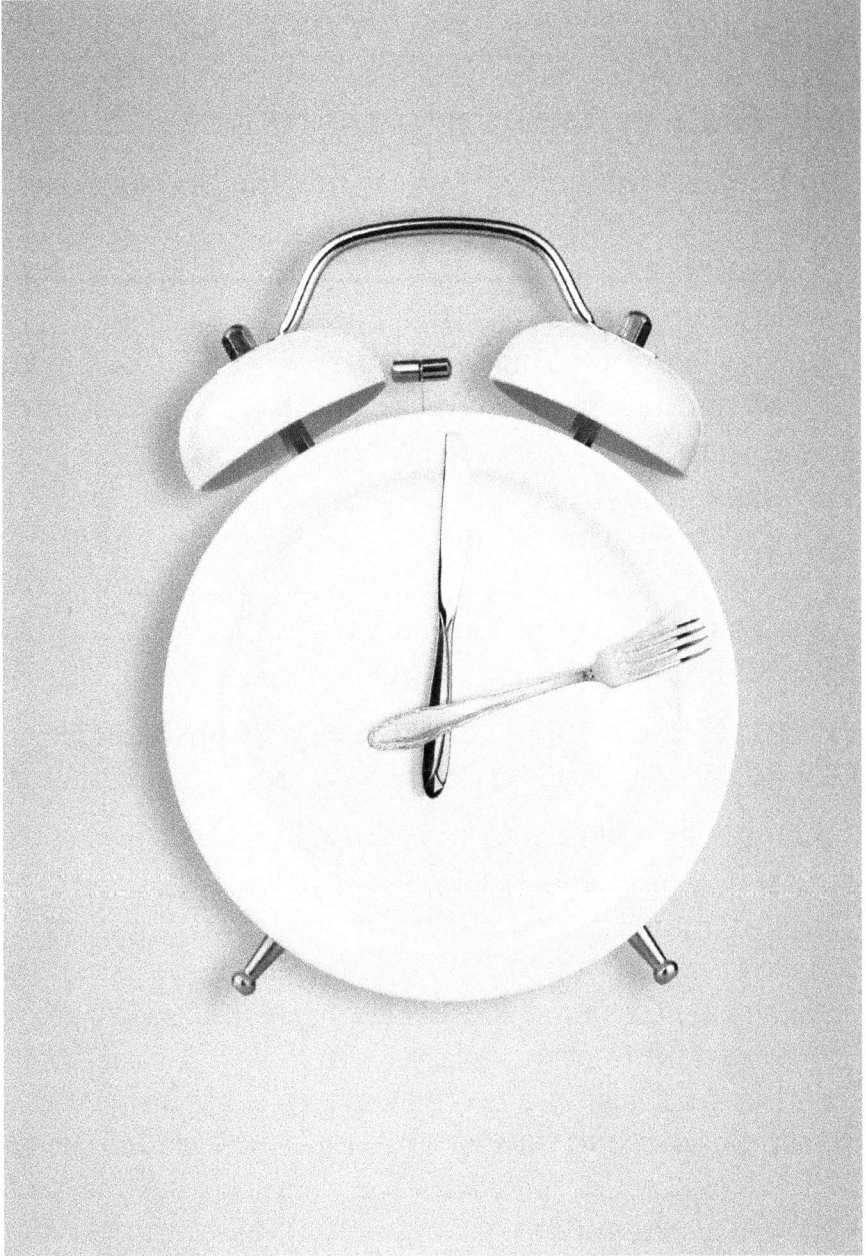

Table of contents

Introduction

Intermittent fasting is one of the most influential health and wellness phenomena in the world right now. People are using it to lose weight, strengthen their wellbeing, and ease their lives. What is Intermittent fasting? Intermittent fasting is a form of eating that switch between fasting and eating times. It doesn't tell you the foods to consume, but rather when you can eat them. In this way, it's more aptly defined as an eating style rather than a diet in common sense. Regular fasting for 24 hours or 16-hour fasts twice a week are two popular intermittent fasting practices.

Humans have practiced fasting since the beginning of time. Supermarkets, refrigerators, and year-round food were not available to ancient hunter-gatherers. They couldn't find anything to consume. As a consequence, humans have adapted to be able to survive for long periods without food.

Fasting has been observed for thousands of years. It has been used to increase focus, prolong life, reduce Alzheimer's disease, prevent insulin tolerance, and even reverse the aging phenomenon.

IF may be achieved in a number of ways, but they often include separating the day or week through feeding and fasting times. The below are the most widely used methods:

- **The 16/8 approach**. The Lean gains procedure also means missing breakfast and reducing everyday feeding to 8 hours, such as 1–9 pm. After that, you swift for 16 hours.

- **Eat-Stop-Eat**: This means fasting for 24 hours once, maybe twice a week, such as not feeding dinner one day to dinner the next.

- **The 5:2 diet:** On two non - consecutive days of the week, you ingest just 500–600 calories, then eat regularly on the remaining five days.

These strategies can help you lose weight by lowering your calorie consumption, as long as you do not compensate by consuming a lot more during the eating hours.

Many individuals find the 16/8 approach to be the easiest, long-term, and quick to adopt. It's also the most well-known.

Intermittent fasting's health advantages are due to improvements in hormone levels, cell structure, and gene expression.

Human growth hormone levels increase while insulin levels decline as you fast. Cells of the body also alter gene expression and activate critical cellular repair processes. Intermittent fasting has a long list of advantages, from weight reduction to improved mental focus, many of which are backed up by science. This eating method is ideal for certain women, but what about those of us who are menopausal or post-menopausal?

When a woman enters her 40s and 50s, her sex hormones spontaneously begin to decrease when the ovaries stop releasing progesterone and estrogen, which causes menstruation to stop. Menopause is described as a woman not having a period for 12 months in a row.

Women may become less receptive to insulin after menopause, so they may have difficulty consuming sugar and processed carbohydrates; such metabolic transition is known as insulin resistance, and it is frequently accompanied by exhaustion and sleeping problems.

Fortunately, people may utilize intermittent fasting to help them navigate the steep roller coaster of menopause. If you're feeling exhaustion, insulin tolerance, or weight gain as a consequence of menopause, you might want to give it a shot.

Intermittent fasting functions on all sides of the calorie calculation. It raises the metabolic rate (calories expended), thereby decreasing the food amount you consume (reduces calorics).

In recent decades, type 2 diabetes has become extremely widespread. Elevated blood sugar levels in the sense of insulin resistance are the most prominent characteristic.

Something that lowers insulin tolerance and protects against type 2 diabetes may help lower blood sugar levels. Intermittent fasting has been found to have significant bencfits for insulin tolerance and to result in a significant decrease in blood sugar levels. Intermittent fasting has been shown to lower fasting blood sugar by 3 to 6 percent and fasting insulin by 20 to 31 percent in human trials.

What should you eat when practicing intermittent fasting? There are no specifications or limitations on what kind of food to consume when practicing intermittent fasting. However, the benefits of IF are unlikely to accompany consistent Big Mac meals.

A well-balanced diet is a secret to losing weight, retaining energy levels, and keeping to the diet. Anyone trying to reduce weight should eat nutrient-dense foods like veggies, fruits, nuts, whole grains, seeds, beans, lean proteins, and dairy.

Our guidelines will be somewhat similar to the foods. We would usually prescribe for better health - unprocessed, high-fiber, whole foods which provide flavor and quality.

To put it another way, if you consume a lot of the foods mentioned in this book, you won't get hungry when fasting.

At the end of your day, the right approach is something that you can handle and maintain over time while not causing any detrimental health effects. This book is a comprehensive guide on Intermittent fasting strategies, how these strategies are beneficial for women over 50, and how they lead to a healthy lifestyle.

Chapter 1: Intermittent Fasting

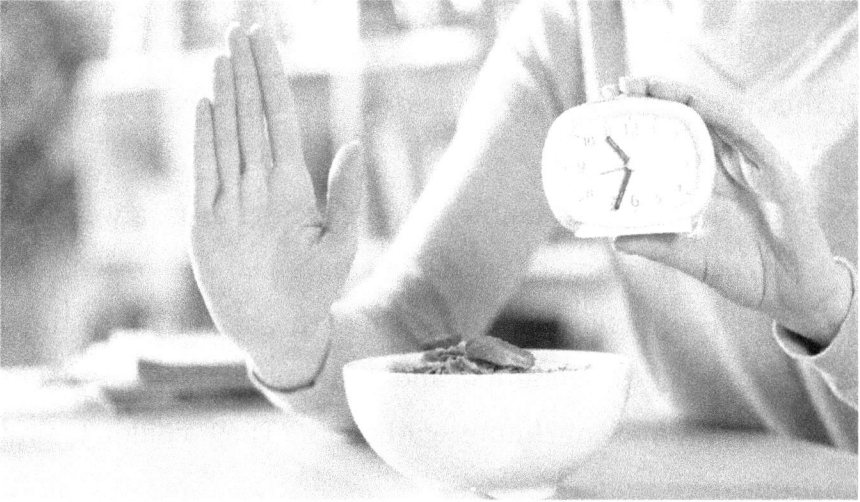

Intermittent fasting is one of the most influential health and wellness phenomena in the world right now. People are using it to lose weight, strengthen their wellbeing, and ease their lives. Several researches has shown to have strong effects on the brain and help one live longer.

This is the comprehensive guide to intermittent fasting for beginners.

1.1 What Is Intermittent Fasting and How Does It Work?

Intermittent fasting is a form of eating that switch between fasting and eating times.

It doesn't tell you the foods to consume, but rather when you can eat them.

In this way, it's more aptly defined as an eating style rather than a diet in common sense.

Regular fasting for 24 hours or 16-hour fasts twice a week are two popular intermittent fasting practices.

Humans have practiced fasting since the beginning of time. Supermarkets, refrigerators, and year-round food were not available to ancient hunter-gatherers. They couldn't find anything to consume.

As a consequence, humans have adapted to be able to survive for long periods without food.

Fasting is, in effect, more normal than consuming 3–4 (or more) meals a day regularly.

Fasting is also observed in Christianity, Islam, Buddhism, and Judaism for spiritual or religious reasons.

1.2 Fasting- History

Fasting has been observed for thousands of years. It has been used to increase focus, prolong life, reduce Alzheimer's disease, prevent insulin tolerance, and even reverse the aging phenomenon. There's a lot to cover here, so we'll open a new segment labeled "Fasting."

Except for what has been overlooked, there is nothing different – Marie Antoinette

And the overlooked weight loss problem is, "When do we eat?" We don't neglect the topic of frequency in any other way. Falling from a 1000-foot building would almost certainly destroy us. Is this, though, the same as 1000 times dropping from a one-foot wall? Certainly not. Despite this, the overall distance travelled is still 1000 miles.

To some extent, all foods raise insulin levels. Eating the right foods will help avoid elevated levels, but it won't help you lower them. Although certain foods are healthier than others, meanwhile all foods raise insulin levels. The trick to avoiding insulin resistance is to maintain extremely low insulin levels on a daily basis. If all foods increase insulin levels, the only option is total voluntary diet abstinence. In a nutshell, the solution we're searching for is fasting.

Fasting

The solution to this perplexing dilemma is found in the tried and tested, not in the new and greatest diet pattern. We should concentrate on ancient medicinal rituals of the past rather than looking for any exotic, never-tried-before diet cure. Fasting is one of the earliest curing rituals known to humanity. About every society and faith on the globe have used this approach.

When the topic of fasting is brought up, everybody rolls their eyes. Is there famine? Is that the solution? No, it's not true. Fasting is an entirely separate phenomenon. The spontaneous lack of food is known as starvation. It's neither planned nor orchestrated. Starving people have no idea where or when their next food will appear. Fasting, on the other side, is the voluntary abstention from eating for moral, nutritional, or other purposes. It's the contrast between attempting suicide and dying of old age. The two words can never be used interchangeably. Fasting may be achieved with as few hours or as many as many months. Fasting is, in certain ways, a function of daily existence. The food that ends the fast – which is performed every day – is referred to as a 'breakfast.'

Fasting is one of the world's oldest and most commonly followed healing rituals. Hippocrates of Cos (c. 460–c. 370 BC) is generally known as the inventor of modern medicine. Fasting and the intake of apple cider vinegar were two of the remedies that he advocated and promoted. To consume while you are sick is to feed your illness, Hippocrates said. Plutarch, an ancient Greek writer and author, repeated these feelings.

"Rather than utilizing medication, better fast today," he said. Plato and his student Aristotle, both ancient Greek philosophers, were enthusiastic advocates of fasting.

Hospital care may be observed in nature, according to the ancient Greeks. When humans, like other species, get ill, they do not feed. Fasting has earned the moniker of the "physician inside." When dogs, cats, and adults are ill, this fasting 'instinct' causes them to become anorexic. This is a feeling that almost everyone has had. Take a minute to remember the last time you were down with the flu. Eating was perhaps the last thing on your mind. As a result, fasting appears to be a universal human impulse in response to various illnesses. Fasting is therefore rooted in human society and is as ancient as history itself.

Fasting was assumed to enhance cognitive abilities by the ancient Greeks. Consider the last time you ate large Thanksgiving dinner. Did you ever feel more energized and centered afterward? Or did you feel drowsy and a bit dopey instead? It's more than definitely the latter. To contend with the enormous influx of calories, blood is redirected to your digestive tract, allowing less blood for the brain. The final effect is a nutritional coma.

Some scholarly giants often advocated fasting. "Fasting is the best cure – the Philip Paracelsus, the inventor of toxicology and is one of the three founders of modern Western medicine (alongside Hippocrates and Galen).

"The greatest of all remedies is resting and fasting," wrote Benjamin Franklin, one of America's founding fathers and a man known for his wide insight of many fields.

Fasting for spiritual reasons is common, and it is a feature of almost every big religion on the planet. Fasting was claimed to have curing abilities by Buddha, the prophet Muhammed, and Jesus Christ. It is often referred to as washing or purification in spiritual terminology, but it is essentially the same thing. Fasting emerged independently from various faiths and traditions, not as a dangerous ritual, but as something that was profoundly, deeply beneficial to the human body and spirit. Food is mostly eaten only in the morning in Buddhism, and adherents fast from noon to the next morning on a regular basis. In addition, numerous water-only fasts for days or even weeks can be experienced.

During the holy month of Ramadan, Muslims fast between sunrise to sunset. Every week on Mondays and Thursdays, the prophet Muhammad urged citizens to fast. Ramadan is the most thoroughly researched of the fasting cycles. Fluids are also prohibited, which sets them apart from many other fasting procedures. They fast and go through a phase of moderate dehydration in addition to fasting. Furthermore, since feeding is allowed prior to sunrise and after sunset, recent research shows that regular caloric intake usually increases during this period. Consuming food before dawn and after sunset seems to counteract some of the positive effects.

As a result, fasting is a concept that has stood the test of time. Fasting is effective, according to the three most famous figures who have ever existed. Do you believe we wouldn't have found this out, say, 1000 years earlier, if this was a dangerous practice?

1.3 Intermittent Fasting Strategies

IF may be achieved in a number of ways, but they often include separating the day or week through feeding and fasting times. You consume very little or none at all during the fasting times. The below are the most widely used methods:

- **The 16/8 approach**. The Lean gains procedure also means missing breakfast and reducing everyday feeding to 8 hours, such as 1–9 pm. After that, you swift for 16 hours.
- **Eat-Stop-Eat**: This means fasting for 24 hours once, maybe twice a week, such as not feeding dinner one day to dinner the next.
- **The 5:2 diet:** On two non - consecutive days of the week, you ingest just 500–600 calories, then eat regularly on the remaining five days.

These strategies can help you lose weight by lowering your calorie consumption, as long as you do not compensate by consuming a lot more during the eating hours.

Many individuals find the 16/8 approach to be the easiest, long-term, and quick to adopt. It's also the most well-known.

1.4 How IF Affects Your Hormones and Cells

Several incidents occur in your body on a cellular and molecular basis as you fast.

To make retained body fat more accessible, the body changes hormone levels, for example.

Essential repair mechanisms and gene expression changes are often initiated by your cells.

When you fast, your body undergoes the following changes:

- **Human Growth Hormone:** Growth hormone levels spike, often by as many as 5-fold. This has a number of advantages, including weight loss and muscle gain.

- **Insulin:** Insulin tolerance increases and insulin levels fall significantly. Lower insulin levels allow stored body fat more available.

- **Cellular repair:** As you fast, your cells tend to repair themselves. Autophagy is a mechanism in which cells ingest and destroy old and damaged proteins that have been collected within them.

- **Gene expression:** There are variations in gene regulation that are linked to survival and disease resistance.

Intermittent fasting's health advantages are due to improvements in hormone levels, cell structure, and gene expression.

Human growth hormone levels increase while insulin levels decline as you fast. Cells of the body also alter gene expression and activate critical cellular repair processes.

1.5 A Very Effective Weight-Loss Tool

The most popular cause for people to attempt intermittent fasting is to lose weight.

- Intermittent fasting will automatically reduce calorie consumption by forcing you to consume less meals.
- Intermittent fasting often alters hormone levels, which aids weight reduction.
- It raises the fat-burning hormone norepinephrine production, reduces insulin, and raises growth hormone levels (noradrenaline).
- Short-term fasting can raise your metabolic rate by 3.6 to 14 percent as a result of these hormonal changes.
- Intermittent fasting induces weight reduction by altering all aspects of the calorie spectrum by assisting you in eating less and burning further calories.
- Intermittent fasting has been shown in experiments to be a very successful weight loss technique.
- This eating pattern will result in 3 to 8% weight loss over 3 to 24 weeks, according to a 2014 analysis report, which is a large amount compared to other weight loss studies.

- According to the same report, people have lost 4 to 7% of their waist circumference, showing a substantial loss of unhealthy belly fat that accumulates around the organs and induces illness.

- In another analysis, intermittent fasting-induced less muscle weakness than the more common form of constant calorie restriction.

- Bear in mind, though, that the key explanation for its popularity is that intermittent fasting allows you to consume fewer calories overall. You do not lose much weight if you binge and consume more through your feeding hours.

1.6 Health Advantages

Intermittent fasting has been studied extensively in both humans and animals.

These findings have shown that it can assist with weight reduction and overall body and brain wellbeing. It may also assist you in living a longer life.

The below are the primary health advantages of intermittent fasting:

- **Weight loss:** As previously mentioned, intermittent fasting will help you lose weight and fat accumulation without intentionally limiting calories.

- **Insulin resistance:** Fasting can help prevent type 2 diabetes by reducing blood sugar levels by 3 to 6% and fasting insulin levels by 20 to 31%.
- **Inflammation:** Several reports indicate a decrease in inflammation markers, a primary driver of many chronic diseases.
- Intermittent fasting has been shown to lower "bad" LDL cholesterol, inflammatory receptors, blood triglycerides, insulin resistance, and blood sugar, both of which are risk factors for cardiac failure.
- Intermittent fasting has been shown in animal research to reduce the risk of cancer.
- **Brain health:** Fasting boosts the brain hormone BDNF, which can help new nerve cells develop. It can also help to prevent Alzheimer's disease.
- **Anti-aging:** Intermittent fasting has been shown to increase the longevity of rats. Fasted rats lived 36 to 83 percent longer, according to studies.

It's important to remember the science is still in its beginnings. The majority of the experiments were limited, short-term, or animal-based. Many concerns remain unanswered in higher-quality human research.

Intermittent fasting has several health advantages for both the body and mind. It will help you lose weight while still lowering the chances of developing type 2 diabetes, cardiac failure, and cancer. It can even assist you in living a longer life.

1.7 Makes Healthy Lifestyle Simpler

Healthy eating is convenient, but it can be challenging to sustain.

One of the most significant barriers is the amount of time and effort to schedule and prepare nutritious meals.

Intermittent fasting will make life simpler, so you don't have to prepare, serve, or clean up as many meals as you would otherwise.

Intermittent fasting is also very common among the life-hacking community, as it enhances your wellbeing while also simplifying your life.

Intermittent fasting has several advantages, one of which is that it allows healthier eating simpler. You'll have less time preparing, cooking, and cleaning up after your meals.

1.8 Who Should Be Cautious of It or Stay Away from It?

Intermittent fasting isn't for everybody.

If you're underweight or even have a record of eating disorders, you can check with a doctor before going on a hard.

It can be downright dangerous in these situations.

Is It Appropriate for Women to Fast?

According to some data, intermittent fasting might not be as effective for women as it is for men.

One research found that it increased insulin response in men but harmed women's blood sugar regulation.

Despite the lack of human research on the topic, studies in rats have shown that intermittent fasting causes female rats to become emaciated, masculinized, infertile, and skip periods.

According to empirical studies, women's menstrual periods ceased after they began doing IF and returned to usual after they continued their former eating routine.

Intermittent fasting can be avoided for women for these purposes.

They should obey their own set of rules, such as gradually introducing the practice and halting quickly if they have any complications, such as amenorrhea (absence of menstruation). Consider delaying intermittent fasting for the time being whether you have pregnancy problems or are planning to conceive. If you're pregnant or breastfeeding, this eating habit is probably not a good one.

Fasting is not recommended for those who are underweight or who with a history of eating disorders. Intermittent fasting can also be detrimental to certain women, according to some facts.

Side Effects and Safety

The most frequent side effect of intermittent fasting is hunger. You, too, can feel tired, and the brain may not do as good as it once did.

This will only be temporary since the body may need time to adjust to the new meal plan.

Before undertaking intermittent fasting, contact the doctor if you've a medical problem.

This is particularly crucial if you:

- You're having trouble controlling your blood sugar.
- You have diabetes.
- Take your medicine as prescribed.
- You have a low blood pressure level.
- Also had an eating problem in the past.
- You're overweight.
- Do you have a diagnosis of amenorrhea?
- You're a mother who's struggling to get pregnant.
- Are breastfeeding or pregnant.

All things considered; intermittent fasting has an excellent safety record. If you're safe and well-nourished generally, going without food for a bit isn't risky.

Hunger is the most frequent side effect of intermittent fasting. Fasting cannot be done without first seeing a specialist if you have a medical problem.

The Frequently Asked Questions

The below are responses to some of the most often asked concerns about intermittent fasting.

- **Am I Allowed to Drink Liquids During My Fast?**

Yes, really. Non-caloric drinks such as water, coffee, and tea are suitable. Coffee cannot be sweetened. Small quantities of milk or cream are probably appropriate. Coffee is particularly helpful during a fast because it suppresses hunger.

- **Isn't Skipping Breakfast Unhealthy?**

No, it's not true. The issue is that most stereotyped breakfast-skippers lead unhealthy lives. The procedure is completely safe if you consume healthy food for the remainder of the day.

- **Am I Allowed to Take Supplements During My Fast?**

Yes, really. Bear in mind, though, that certain supplements, such as fat-soluble vitamins, can function best if taken with food.

- **Can I Exercise When I'm Fasting?**

Fasted workouts are perfectly acceptable. Before a fasted exercise, certain people consider taking branched-chain amino acids (BCAAs).

- **Is it True That Fasting Induces Muscle Loss?**

Both weight reduction strategies will result in muscle loss; that's why it's important to raise weights and consume plenty of protein. Intermittent fasting produces less muscle weakness than normal calorie restriction, according to one report.

- **Can Fasting Make Metabolism Slow Down?**

No, studies indicate that fasting for a brief period boosts metabolism. Fasting for three or four days, on the other hand, will slow down metabolism.

- **Should Children Be Pushed to Fast?**

It's probably not a good idea to let your child fast.

1.9 Getting Stated

You've already undergone a lot of extended fasting in your life. If you've ever eaten dinner but slept late the next day and didn't feed before noon, you've fasted for 16 hours or more.

This is how some people feed naturally. In the morning, they do not feel hungry.

Many individuals consider the 16/8 approach to be the most straightforward and long-lasting method of intermittent fasting; you may want to start with. If you like fasting and feel healthy while doing so, you might progress to more extreme fasts such as 24-hour fasts 1 to 2 times a week (that is Eat-Stop-Eat) or just consuming 500–600 calories 1 to 2 days a week (that is 5:2 diet).

Another choice is to easily fast anytime possible — miss meals when you aren't hungry or don't have time to prepare them.

To reap at least any of the rewards, you don't need to implement a formal intermittent fasting schedule.

Experiment with various methods before you discover one that you like and works into your routine.

It's best to begin with, the 16/8 approach and work your way up to longer fasts later. It's crucial to try out different methods before you discover one that fits you.

1.10 Should You Give This a Try?

Anyone does not need to practice intermittent fasting.

It's only one of the lifestyle changes that will help you live a healthier life. The most critical things to concentrate on are always eating real food, exercising, and getting enough sleep.

If you don't like the thought of fasting, you should easily disregard this bok and proceed to do what you want.

When it comes to diet, there is no such thing as a one-size-fits-all approach. The safest lifestyle for you is one that you can maintain with time.

Few individuals reap from intermittent fasting, and others do not. You can only figure out which party you belong to by trying it out.

Fasting may be an effective strategy for losing weight and improving your fitness if you like it and believe it to be a sustainable form of eating.

Chapter 2: Intermittent Fasting Benefits For 50 Years Old Women

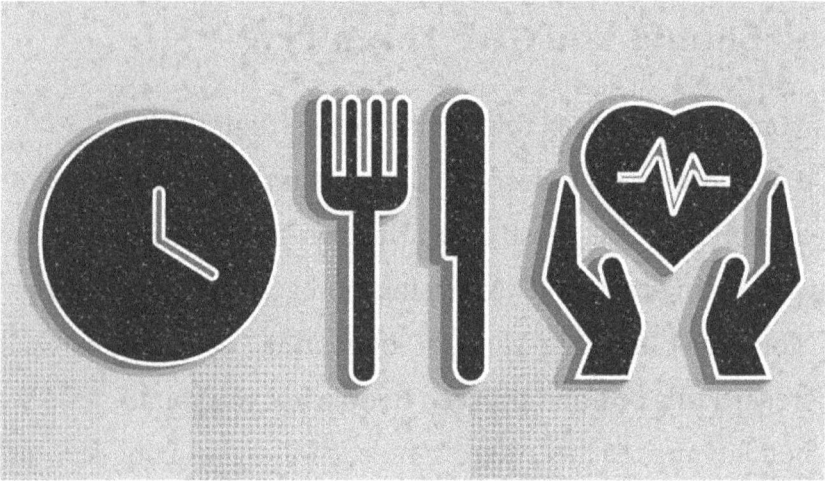

Intermittent fasting is the eating practice under which you alternate between eating and fasting patterns. Intermittent fasting can be done in a variety of ways, such as the 5:2 or 16/8 techniques.

Numerous researches has shown that it can have significant health and cognitive effects. Here are some of the health effects of prolonged fasting that have been clinically proven.

2.1 Intermittent fasting and loss of stubborn body fat

Anyone who has ever been on a strict diet and reached single-digit body fat levels is familiar with the problem: stubborn fat. Despite extensive workout and drastically diminished calorie consumption, a moderate amount of body fat also provides resistance. Most of them soon realize that in order to eliminate these fat deposits, they would have to sacrifice a significant amount of weight.

Will Intermittent Fasting, on the other hand, aid in the loss of stubborn fat?

Stubborn fat refers to fat deposits that the body refuses to release.

As we previously said, intermittent fasting will help you avoid the difficulties of losing stubborn body fats.

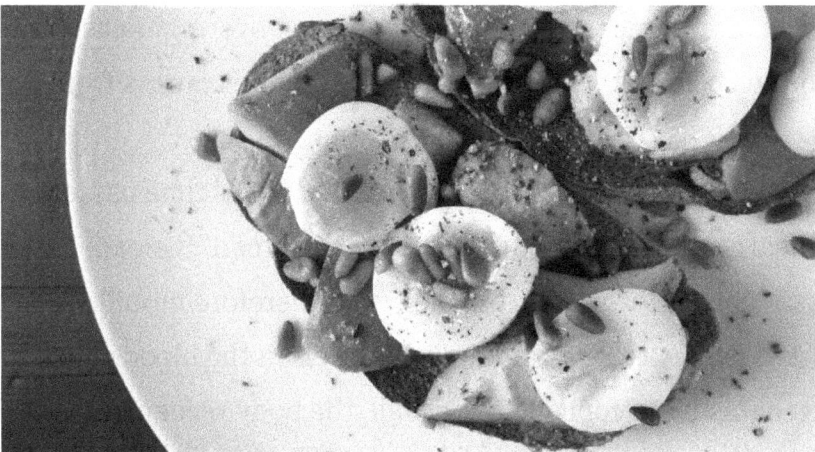

What Is the Definition of Stubborn Body Fat?

The word "stubborn body fat" applies to the body parts that hold the most fat. In general, these regions are the lower abdomen region and the lower back in males and the lower body in women. It's very difficult to lose weight in these regions.

So what is it that renders these places so obstinate? Let's take a peek at how fat is mobilized and get a better understanding of this. Are you prepared?

The insulin level and fatty acid content (in the blood) rise after a meal. It is in saturated form where there is no fat burning. The body gets the energy it needs in the hours after that by oxidizing (metabolizing) glucose.

The respiratory quotient is one way to calculate this (RQ). A value of 1.0 indicates pure carb metabolism (storage mode), while a value of 0.7 refers to enhanced fatty acid metabolism (lipid metabolism). This implies for the RQ in the form of intermittent fasting: The RQ is between 0.95 to 1.0 in 1.5–2 hours after a meal. The quotient after an overnight easy range from 0.82 to 0.85, and after a 16-hour lent, it ranges from 0.72 to 0.8.

Both the insulin concentration and RQ drop as time passes after a meal and the body's nutrients are consumed. Instead, a trend has occurred toward fat-burning (and therefore mobilization of stored fat). Fatty acids and insulin levels in the blood cause this mechanism. As concentrations fall, the body recognizes an energy shortfall and enhances catecholamine secretion as a consequence (epinephrine and norepinephrine).

Catecholamines in the blood adhere to fat cell receptors. These receptors may be thought of as a "lock" symbolically. Neurotransmitters and Hormones are the keys that fit into these locks, causing a response. In this situation, catecholamines cause (activate) fat mobilization by activating the HSL "hormone-sensitive lipase," for short, which then produces fat from the individual cell, which could then be burned (metabolized).

The main distinction between natural fat and stubborn fat deposits is as follows. Beta-2 receptors are far more abundant in normal adipose tissue than alpha-2 receptors.

Beta-2 receptors are known as the 'gas pedal' for reducing fat. Meanwhile, alpha-2 receptors mostly behave like an auto brake You don't have to go too far into the physiology to imagine these two receptors like this.

How simple it is to burn fat in different body areas is determined by the interaction between alpha-2 and beta-2 receptors. When the fat of a body area has many beta-2 receptors compared to alpha-2 receptors, "light" or "simple" fat burning happens, while chronic fat pads have several numbers of alpha-2 receptors compared to beta-2 receptors.

In the region of the hips and thighs, women have up to 9 times the number of alpha-2 receptors compared to beta-2 receptors, according to Lyle's book.

Body Fat Reduction

How does intermittent fasting burn stubborn fat more effectively than most diets? The beta-2 receptors should now be programmed, while the alpha-2 receptors must be deactivated to metabolize persistent fat deposits. The processes that allow for intermittent fasting are as follows.

Catecholamine levels rise as you fast.

Fasting improves subcutaneous blood supply in the abdominal region, allowing catecholamines to penetrate this area more easily (and, consequently, dock to the cell receptors of fat).

Fasting prevents a2 receptors due to low insulin levels. More time spent in the "fast window" ensures more fat can be extracted from stubborn areas. Now you could be thinking, "Why don't I just follow a low-carb diet to maintain my insulin levels low?" However, triglycerides (fats) block hormone-sensitive lipase in the same way as insulin does.

According to research, the optimal fat-burning condition is achieved after 12-18 hours of fasting. This time can be called the "golden era" for the recruitment of stubborn fat due to the high catecholamines level, the elevated subcutaneous blood supply in the stubborn fat areas, and a low insulin level for the necessary alpha 2 receptor inhibition.

Let it be more clarified by an optimal condition of fat burning in a few words: The oxidation of FFA (free fatty acids) – in various locations between both the fasting state and after three consecutive days of fasting – has been studied. The amount of burned fatty acids has shifted in relation to body fat's total metabolism, while FFA oxidation has risen with the length of fasting time.

The oxidation of subcutaneous FFA rises dramatically over short durations. This is also a long way of suggesting that you burn the fat and nothing else. Fat deposits will only mobilize fat in a latent, normal-weight human for 14–20 hours after a 600kcal meal. In actual life, this condition should be possible to achieve in 12–18 hours.

Fat burning begins to rise after this time window (14–20 hours). Conversely, this isn't the sort of fat we choose to get rid of. Oxidation of intramuscular fat rises dramatically between 10 to 30 hours, but there is no rise in subcutaneous fat deposits.

If the fasting window is extended so long, the dermal depots can't keep up with the body's amount of energy, so there is a limited degree of benefit and disadvantage. Rather long cycles of fasting are not conducive to the reduction of stubborn body fat, thus optimizing muscle preservation, leading to the elevated rate of gluconeogenesis (protein saccharification) and the resulting possibility of the catabolic condition of the muscles.

Real Life Vs. Science

Investing Critically, Readers can now question if getting rid of stubborn fat necessitates some unique methods. After all, several individuals have already reached "lean" status without utilizing intermittent fasting or other methods like those mentioned by Lyle McDonald. Isn't it just about lowering the body fat level as much as possible? Isn't it likely that you'll lose the stubborn fat anyway?

Can a 3500 kcal weekly deficit in a commonly practiced diet against an equivalent deficit in an intermittent fasting diet create a difference in regional fat loss (assuming all other variables remain constant)? The statement is limited to theoretical implications and practical observations.

2.2 Menopause and intermittent fasting

IF is one of the most common methods for losing weight and improving general wellbeing. It entails going without food for most of the day and consuming all of the meals in a short period.

Intermittent fasting has a long list of advantages, from weight reduction to improved mental focus, many of which are backed up by science. This eating method is ideal for certain women, but what about those of us who are menopausal or post-menopausal?

When a woman enters her 40s and 50s, her sex hormones spontaneously begin to decrease when the ovaries stop releasing progesterone and estrogen, which causes menstruation to stop. Menopause is described as a woman not having a period for 12 months in a row, but amenorrhea is far from the only symptom of the change.

Hot flashes, anxiety, vaginal dryness, brain fog, reduced libido, chills, exhaustion, mood swings, an elevated likelihood of heart problems, and night sweats are some of the signs of menopause, which can range from individual to individual. There is often a noticeable difference in metabolism with certain people, which usually speeds down when estrogen and progesterone levels get out of control, causing weight gain.

Women may become less receptive to insulin after menopause, so they may have difficulty consuming sugar and processed carbohydrates; such metabolic transition is known as insulin resistance, and it is frequently accompanied by exhaustion and sleeping problems.

Many people find menopause a frightening period in their lives; they can no longer recognize their bodies, and symptoms including sudden brain fog and weight gain may cause anxicty, confusion, rage, stress, and depression.

Fortunately, people may utilize intermittent fasting to help them navigate the steep roller coaster of menopause. If you're feeling exhaustion, insulin tolerance, or weight gain as a consequence of menopause, you might want to give it a shot.

Weight gain has been found to be aided by intermittent fasting. Fasting improves insulin control and makes the body absorb sugar and carbohydrates more efficiently, lowering the risk of heart failure, diabetes, and other metabolic diseases. Fasting has been proven to increase self-esteem, minimize distress and tension, and encourage more beneficial psychological improvements. Fasting has been shown in animal research to help shield brain cells from trauma, clean out waste products, restore and improve their performance.

When you have a schedule in place, intermittent fasting isn't all that complicated. Simply set an eating window that fits you, such as noon to 8 pm, and make sure you consume enough of the calories at that time. Outside of that window, you must fast. However, you are allowed to drink water and non-caloric beverages such as tea or coffee. The 16:8 form of fasting entails fasting for 16 hours a day and feeding for just 8 hours a day; it is one of the most basic intermittent fasting processes to adopt. Intermittent fasting is simple and adaptable; some people begin with shorter fasting times, such as 14:10 (14 hours of fasting accompanied by a 10-hour consuming window), and steadily extend the fasting duration before they achieve the target of 16:8. You should experiment with various fasting routines and see what fits and sounds better for you because of the simplicity and stability.

Although intermittent fasting is a wonderful tool for most people to better relieve the effects of menopause, it is not for all.

Those that have adrenal exhaustion or a chronic condition do not choose to add an intermittent fasting method into their schedules.

Much intermittent practice fasting should pay attention to how they feel throughout the fasting cycle; if you get tired, sluggish, or sick when fasting, it might be better to either reduce the fasting period or avoid attempting intermittent fasting altogether. You also don't have to fast daily; you can fast once a week or even a couple of days a week. To prevent risks and guarantee that every diet or lifestyle modification is right for you, it's also a good idea to speak with a qualified and licensed medical practitioner first.

Menopause is a tough period for most people, but by making the correct food and behavioral adjustments, you can better control the effects and remain fit, comfortable, and safe even when the hormones try to change it and finally exit the building.

2.3 Intermittent fasting alters gene, hormone, and cell function

When you don't feed for a bit, the body goes through a lot of shifts.

To render accumulated body fat more available, the body, for example, initiates essential cellular repair mechanisms and adjusts hormone levels.

—

Here are some of the physiological modifications that arise during fasting:

- **Insulin levels:** Insulin levels in the blood decrease dramatically, facilitating fat burning.
- **Human growth hormone:** Growth hormone levels in the blood will rise by up to 5-fold. Increased amounts of this hormone help with weight loss and muscle growth, among other things.
- **Cellular repair:** The body initiates critical cellular repair procedures, such as removing waste from cells.
- **Gene expression:** There are positive variations in several genes and molecules linked to survival and disease prevention.

These improvements in hormones, gene expression, and cell structure are linked to many of the advantages of intermittent fasting.

Insulin levels decrease, and human growth hormone levels rise as you fast. Your cells also activate critical cellular repair mechanisms and alter the expression of genes.

2.4 Weight Loss and Belly Fat Loss Can Be Achieved by Intermittent Fasting

Many people who experiment with intermittent fasting do so in order to reduce weight.

In general, extended fasting causes you to consume less meals. You might require fewer calories if you compensate for consuming even more during the other meals.

Intermittent fasting often improves hormone function, which aids weight reduction.

Reduced insulin levels, higher productivity of growth hormone levels, and higher noradrenaline (norepinephrine) levels all help the body break down fat and use it for energy.

As a result, short-term fasting boosts the metabolic rate by 3.6 to 14%, allowing you to eat even more cal.

Intermittent fasting, in other words, functions on all sides of the calorie calculation. It raises the metabolic rate (calories expended), thereby decreasing the food amount you consume (reduces calories).

According to a 2014 study of the clinical literature, intermittent fasting will result in weight loss of 3 to 8 percent over 3 to 24 weeks. This is a massive amount.

The participants have lost four to 7 percent of their waist circumference, indicating that they lost a lot of belly fat, the disease-causing fat in the abdominal cavity.

Intermittent fasting showed fewer muscle loss than prolonged calorie restriction, according to a review report.

When it is said and done, intermittent fasting may be a very effective weight-loss strategy.

Intermittent fasting allows you to consume fewer calories while marginally increasing your metabolism. It's a powerful weapon for losing weight and belly fat.

2.5 Insulin Resistance May Be Reduced by Intermittent Fasting, Lowering the Risk of Developing Type 2 Diabetes

In recent decades, type 2 diabetes has become extremely widespread.

Elevated blood sugar levels in the sense of insulin resistance are the most prominent characteristic.

Something that lowers insulin tolerance and protects against type 2 diabetes may help lower blood sugar levels.

Intermittent fasting has also been found to have significant benefits for insulin tolerance and to result in a significant decrease in blood sugar levels.

Intermittent fasting has been shown to lower fasting blood sugar by 3 to 6 percent and fasting insulin by 20 to 31 percent in human trials.

Intermittent fasting often prevented diabetic rats from kidney injury, which is one of the most serious consequences of diabetes.

This means that intermittent fasting could be very beneficial for individuals at risk of having type 2 diabetes. There might, still, be certain gender disparities. According to one report, during a 22-day intermittent fasting regimen, women's blood sugar management actually deteriorated. At least in men, intermittent fasting will reduce insulin resistance and aid in lowering blood sugar levels.

2.6 Intermittent Fasting Can Lower Inflammation in the Body and Oxidative Stress

Oxidative stress is one of the factors that contribute to aging and the development of several chronic diseases. It entails reactive molecules such as free radicals interacting with and destroying other essential molecules (such as protein and DNA). Intermittent fasting has been shown in some trials to improve the body's tolerance to oxidative stress.

In addition, research indicates that intermittent fasting may help combat inflammation, which is a major cause of a variety of diseases.

Intermittent fasting has been shown in studies to decrease inflammation in the body and oxidative stress. This should help prevent aging and the onset of a variety of diseases.

2.7 Intermittent Fasting Might Be Good for The Heart

Heart attack is still the world's leading cause of death.

Various health indicators (also regarded as "risk factors") have been linked to an elevated or reduced cardiac failure risk.

Intermittent fasting was shown to improve total and LDL cholesterol, blood pressure, inflammation receptors, blood sugar levels, and blood triglycerides, among other risk factors.

However, a large amount of this is focused on animal science. Before any decisions can be developed, further research on the impact on humans' heart health is needed.

Intermittent fasting has been shown in studies to improve cholesterol levels, blood pressure, inflammatory receptors, and triglycerides, all of which contribute to heart disease.

2.8 Various Cellular Repair Mechanisms Are Triggered by Intermittent Fasting

When you fast, the cells in the body start a process called autophagy, a cellular waste removal process.

Broken and damaged proteins that accumulate within cells over time are broken down and metabolized by the cells.

Increased autophagy could protect against cancer and Alzheimer's disease, among other diseases.

Fasting activates the autophagy metabolic system, which eliminates waste from cells.

2.9 Intermittent Fasting Has Been Linked to A Lower Risk of Cancer

Cancer is a horrific disease that is marked by uncontrollable cell development.

Fasting has been found to have a variety of biochemical advantages, including a decreased incidence of cancer.

Despite the lack of human trials, encouraging data from animal studies suggests that intermittent fasting can help to prevent cancer.

Fasting minimized multiple side effects of chemotherapy in cancer patients, according to some evidence.

In animal research, intermittent fasting has been shown to better suppress cancer. In humans, one study found that it would eliminate chemotherapy side effects.

2.10 Intermittent Fasting Is Beneficial to The Brain

What is healthy for the body is frequently always good for the brain.

Intermittent fasting increases the number of biochemical characteristics that are linked to brain health.

Reduced oxidative stress, inflammation, blood sugar levels, and insulin tolerance are all part of this.

Intermittent fasting has been shown in rats' experiments to accelerate the development of new nerve cells, which could improve brain activity.

It often boosts a brain hormone known as BDNF (brain-derived neurotrophic factor), whose deficiency has been related to depression and other neurological issues.

Intermittent fasting has also been found to guard against brain injury caused by strokes in animals.

Therefore, Intermittent fasting can have significant health benefits for the brain. It has the potential to promote the development of new neurons while still protecting the brain from injury.

2.11 Intermittent Fasting May Aid in The Prevention of Alzheimer's Disease

The most prevalent neurodegenerative disorder in the world is Alzheimer's disease.

Since there is no treatment for Alzheimer's disease, stopping it from developing in the first place is crucial.

According to a rat report, intermittent fasting can postpone the onset of Alzheimer's disease or minimize its intensity.

According to a series of case studies, a dietary intervention that involved regular short-term fasts substantially reduced Alzheimer's symptoms in nine out of ten patients.

According to animal research, fasting may also guard against some neurodegenerative disorders, such as Huntington's and Parkinson's disease.

However, further human testing is needed.

2.12 Intermittent Fasting Can Help You Live Longer by Increasing Your Life Span

One of the most intriguing aspects of intermittent fasting is the potential to prolong life expectancy.

Intermittent fasting increases longevity in rats in the same manner as constant calorie restriction would.

The results of some of these experiments were very dramatic. One of them found that rats who fasted every other day survived 83 percent longer than rats who didn't fast.

Intermittent fasting has been very common among the anti-aging community, despite the fact that it has yet to be demonstrated in humans.

With the effects of intermittent fasting for metabolism and a variety of health indicators, it's easy to see how it might aid live a longer and happier life.

Chapter 3: Get Started with Intermittent Fasting

3.1 What Are the Healthiest Intermittent Fasting Foods?

We include items that we believe would be beneficial to our readers. Please contact a health practitioner before undertaking any major dietary adjustments to ensure that it is the right choice for you.

Intermittent fasting makes quite an uproar in the overpopulated world of dieting, despite the phrase "fasting" appears quite ominous. A fair amount of evidence (albeit with small sample sizes) shows that the diet can help people lose weight and control their blood sugar levels. Maybe the appeal stems from the lack of diet restrictions: you can consume what you want, but not exactly when you want.

However, it's still necessary to consider what's at stake. Should you be breaking your fast with ice cream pints and bags of chips? Very likely not. That's why we've compiled a collection of the best things to eat on an IF diet.

What Should You Eat?

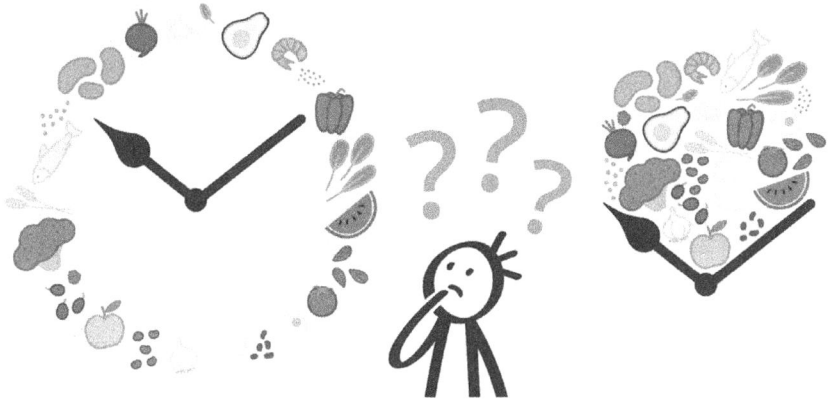

There are no specifications or limitations on what kind of food to consume when practicing intermittent fasting. However, the benefits of IF are unlikely to accompany consistent Big Mac meals.

A well-balanced diet is a secret to losing weight, retaining energy levels, and keeping to the diet.

Anyone trying to reduce weight should eat nutrient-dense foods like veggies, fruits, nuts, whole grains, seeds, beans, lean proteins, and dairy.

Our guidelines will be somewhat similar to the foods. We would usually prescribe for better health - unprocessed, high-fiber, whole foods which provide flavor and quality.

To put it another way, if you consume a lot of the foods mentioned below, you won't get hungry when fasting.

- **Water**

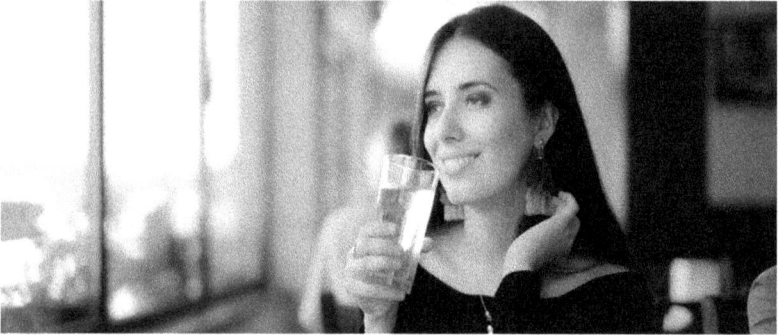

Well, so this isn't a snack, but it's crucial for surviving IF. Water is important for the protection of almost all of your body's main organs. Avoiding this as part of the fast will be stupid. Your lungs play a critical role in keeping you safe. The amount of water that each individual can drink depends on their gender, height, weight, exercise level, and environment. However, the color of the urine is a strong indicator. For all times, you like it to be pale yellow. Dehydration, which may induce headaches, nausea, and lightheadedness, is shown by dark yellow urine. When you combine it with a lack of calories, you have a formula for catastrophe or, at the very worst, really dark pee. If plain water doesn't appeal to you, try adding a splash of lemon juice, several mint leaves, or cucumber slices to it.

- **Avocado**

Eating the highest-calorie fruit when attempting to lose weight can appear counterintuitive. On the other hand, avocados can hold you complete through even the most stringent fasting times due to its high unsaturated fat content.

Unsaturated fats, according to studies, help hold the body healthy even though you don't feel hungry. Your body sends out signals that it doesn't need to go into emergency hunger mode because it has enough calories. And if you're starving in the midst of a fasting time, unsaturated fats hold these symptoms are running much longer.

Another research showed that using half an avocado with your lunch will help you stay full for hours longer than it would be if you don't consume the green, mushy fruit.

- **Seafood And Fish**

There's an explanation why the American Dietary Guidelines recommend two or three 4-oz. portions of fish every week.

In contrast to being rich in beneficial fats and protein, it is also high in vitamin D.

And if you like to feed at short window periods, don't you want to get more nutritious bang for the buck when you do? You'll never run out of ways to prepare fish since there are too many options.

- **Cruciferous Veggies**

The f-word — fiber — is abundant in foods like brussels sprouts, cauliflower, and broccoli.

It's important to consume fiber-rich foods regularly to keep you regular and ensure that your poop runs smoothly.

Fiber will also help you feel full, which is beneficial if you won't feed for another 16 hours. Cruciferous vegetables will also help you avoid cancer.

- **Potatoes**

White foods aren't all evil.

Potatoes were found to be one of the most nutritious foods in 1990s research.

a reliable source, a 2012 study showed that using potatoes in a balanced diet can aid weight loss. (Sorry, but potato chips and French fries don't count.)

- **Legumes And Beans**

On the IF diet, your favorite chili topping might be your best pal.

Food, especially carbohydrates, provides energy for physical exercise. We're not suggesting you go crazy with carbohydrates, so including low-calorie carbs like legumes and beans in your diet can't hurt. This will help you stay alert through your fasting period.

Furthermore, ingredients like black beans, chickpeas, lentils, and peas have been proven to help people lose weight, particularly though they aren't on a diet.

- **Probiotics**

What do the tiny critters in your stomach want to eat the most? Both consistency and variety are essential. If they're starving, this means they're not comfortable. And if your stomach isn't comfortable, you may notice any unpleasant side effects, such as constipation.

Add probiotic-rich ingredients to the diet, such as kefir, kombucha, and sauerkraut, to combat this unpleasantness.

- **Berries**

These smoothie classics are packed with vitamins and minerals. That's not even the most exciting aspect. People who ate a lot of flavonoids, such as those used in strawberries and blueberries, had lower BMI rises over 14 years than individuals who didn't eat berries, according to a 2016 report.

- **Eggs**

One big egg has 6.24 g of protein and takes just minutes to prepare. And, particularly when you are eating less, having as many proteins as possible is critical for staying full and building muscle.

Men who had an egg breakfast rather than a bagel have been less hungry and ate less during the day, according to a 2010 survey.

To put it another way, if you're looking for something else to do during your fast, why not hard-boil a bunch of eggs? And, when the time is perfect, you should eat them.

- **Nuts**

While nuts are higher in cal than many other snacks, they do have something that most snacks do not: healthy fats.

Even don't be thinking about calories! According to a 2012 report, a 1-oz. serving of almonds (roughly 23 nuts) contains 20% less calories than the label claims.

According to the report, chewing does not fully break down the cell walls of almonds, which keeps a part of the nut safe and prevents it from being absorbed by the body through digestion. As a result, eating almonds might not make as much of a difference in your regular calorie intake as you would think.

- **Whole Grains**

Dieting and carbohydrate use tend to fall under two distinct categories. This isn't always the case, as you'll be glad to learn. Since whole grains are high in fiber and nutrition, a small amount would keep you satisfied for a long time.

So get out of your comfort zone and try bulgur, farro, spelt, amaranth, kamut, millet, freekeh, or sorghum.

Caution

Tiredness, headaches, and irritability are all side effects of IF. If you do not drink enough water during your fast, you could get dehydrated.

According to rat studies, IF can also lead to infertility. Athletes will often notice that their workouts' pacing in the energy cycle causes them to break down muscle rather than develop it.

Fasting/feasting is, therefore, theoretically impractical in the long run since it can contribute to binge consumption during feasting hours, which would undermine any weight-loss efforts. If you consume the foods mentioned above during yo-yo dieting, they cannot have the nutritious benefits you want. When the body is stressed due to not consuming enough calories, it cannot use the foods you can consume to their maximum potential.

The long-term weight reduction that is steady and durable may be better. Since there isn't any literature on IF right now, the long-term consequences remain largely unknown.

Before starting IF, speak to a dietitian or nutritionist to make sure it's right for you.

IF isn't an invitation to binge feed; it's a time to be selective with what you eat. And whether you fast or not, the ingredients in this book should be a big part of your diet.

3.2 Foods to Consume and Prevent During Intermittent Fasting

Eat vegetables and fruits when on an intermittent fasting diet and stop sugary and processed snacks.

Intermittent Fasting entails alternating between feeding and fasting times.

Intermittent fasting, according to proponents, is a healthy and easy way to reduce weight and boost your fitness. They say it's simpler to stick to than other diets and that it has greater versatility than conventional calorie-restricted diets. "Rather than relying on permanent dietary restriction, intermittent fasting is a way of lowering calories by limiting one's consumption for many days per week and only consuming normally the rest of the days," says Lisa Jones, a licensed dietitian in Philadelphia.

It's crucial to remember that intermittent fasting is a concept rather than a strict diet.

According to Anna Kippen, a licensed dietitian in Cleveland, 'IF is an umbrella word for the eating pattern that involves cycles of non-fasting and fasting over fixed periods. "Intermittent fasting comes in a variety of ways."

Time-restricted feeding is one of the more common methods. It recommends feeding only for eight hours a day and fasting for the next 16 hours. "It will help us lose weight while still allowing our gut and hormones to relax between meals throughout our 'fast," says Kippen.

The 5:2 strategy, in which you eat normally and healthily for five days a week, is another common solution. You only eat one meal a day on the remaining two days of the week, which can be between 500 and 700 calories. "This helps our bodies to relax while still growing the number of calories we eat during the week," Kippen explains.

IF has been linked to weight reduction, increased cholesterol, blood sugar regulation, and reduced inflammation in research.

According to a report released, prolonged fasting has broad-spectrum effects for multiple health problems, such as obesity, cardiovascular disease, diabetes, tumors, and neurologic disorders.

According to Ryan Maciel, a dietitian, "whatever type of intermittent fasting you want, it's crucial to adhere the same basic nutrition concepts to intermittent fasting as to other healthier eating plans."

"In reality, these (principles) might be much more relevant when you're going without food for longer periods, which may contribute to overeating in certain people," Maciel says.

If you are on an intermittent fasting plan, here are few guidelines to follow:

- Eat items that are minimally refined the majority of the time.

- Have a variety of lean protein, vegetables, fruits, smart carbs, and good fats in your diet.
- Cook delectable, tasty recipes that you can enjoy.
- Slowly and mindfully eat your meals till you're pleased.

Diets based on intermittent fasting do not include complex menus. However, adhering to healthy eating practices, there are some items that should be consumed and those that should be avoided.

On an extended fasting diet, you can consume the following three foods:

- Fruits
- Lean proteins
- Vegetables

Lean Proteins

According to Maciel, eating lean protein makes you fuller for longer than most diets and helps you sustain or gain muscle. Here are five protein sources that are both lean and healthy:

- Plain Greek yogurt
- Tofu and tempeh
- Chicken breast
- Fish and shellfish
- Beans, lentils, and peas

Fruits

Intermittent fasting, as every other meal plan, necessitates the consumption of high-nutrient foods. Vitamins, phytonutrients (plant nutrients), fiber, and minerals are commonly found in vegetables and fruits. These vitamins, minerals, and nutrients may reduce cholesterol, blood sugar regulation, and bowel health. Another advantage is the reduced calorie content of fruits and vegetables.

Here are ten nutritious fruits to eat while fasting intermittently:

- Apricots
- Apples
- Blackberries
- Blueberries
- Peaches
- Cherries
- Plums
- Pears
- Watermelon
- Oranges

Vegetables

Vegetables will help you stick to your intermittent fasting plan. A diet high in leafy greens has been shown to lower the risk of heart failure, Type 2 diabetes, cognitive impairment, cancer, and other diseases.

Here are 6 vegetables that will be beneficial to use in a balanced intermittent eating plan:

- Spinach

- Kale
- Cabbage
- Chard
- Arugula
- Collard greens

Foods To Stay Away From

Certain ingredients cannot be consumed as part of the IF protocol. Avoid foods that are rich in fat, salt, and sugar and are high in calories. "They won't satisfy you after a fast, and they might even leave you hungry," Maciel warns. "They still don't have anything in the way of nutrients."

Avoid the following foods if you choose to stick to an intermittent diet plan:

- Chips for a snack
- Microwave Popcorn

Foods containing a lot of added sugar should also be prevented. According to Maciel, sugar in packaged foods and beverages is deprived of nutrients and contributes to sweet, hollow calories, which is not what you want while you're intermittently fasting. "Because sugar metabolizes too quickly, they'll leave you hungry," he adds.

3.3 List of Foods for Intermittent Fasting

Don't know what to feed while you're fasting intermittently? The definitive IF food list, backed by science, can help you get the best out of your weight loss path.

It's difficult to know what to eat during IF. This is because IF is a dietary habit rather than a diet. With this in mind, we have created an IF food list that will keep you well as you lose weight. The IF program teaches you when to eat, so it doesn't tell you what ingredients you should eat. Lack of consistent dietary advice can offer the feeling that you can consume anything you want. Others may have difficulty selecting the "appropriate" foods and beverages as a result of this.

These not only thwart your weight-loss plans but also increase your chances of being malnourished or over nourished.

3.4 How to Choose the Most Appropriate Foods

It's more essential to eat healthily through intermittent fasting than it is to lose weight quickly. As a result, choosing nutrient-dense foods like vegetables, lean proteins, good fats, and fruits is vital.

The food list for intermittent fasting should include:

For Protein

Protein has an RDA (Recommended Dietary Allowance) of 0.8 g per kg of body weight. Depending on your fitness objectives and level of exercise, your needs may vary.

Protein aids weight loss by lowering calorie consumption, rising satiety, and speeding up metabolism.

Increased protein consumption often aids muscle growth when paired with resistance training. Muscle burns more cal than fat, so getting more muscle in the body improves your metabolism. According to a recent report, having more strength in the legs will help healthier men shed belly fat.

The Intermittent fasting food list for the proteins include:

- Seafood
- Eggs
- Dairy products, for example, yogurt, cheese, and milk
- Beans and legumes
- Seeds and nuts
- Whole grains
- Soy

For Carbs

Carbohydrates can account for 45 - 65 percent of the daily cal, as per the American Dietary Guidelines

Carbohydrates are the body's primary supply of energy. Protein and fat are the remaining two. Carbohydrates come in several ways. Ber, starch, and sugar are the most well-known.

Carbs have a negative reputation for promoting weight gain. On the other hand, Carbs are not necessarily made equal, and they are not always fattening.

The type and quantity of carbohydrates you consume determine whether or not you put on weight.

Be sure you consume diets rich in fiber and starch but lower in sugar.

According to a 2015 report, consuming 30 g of beer per day will help you lose weight, raise your blood glucose levels, and lower your blood pressure.

The Intermittent fasting food list for the carbs include:

- Beetroots
- Sweet potatoes
- Oats
- Quinoa
- Brown rice
- Mangoes
- Bananas
- Berries
- Apples
- Pears
- Kidney beans
- Carrots
- Avocado
- Brussels sprouts

- Broccoli
- Chia seeds
- Almonds
- Chickpeas

For Fats

Fats should account for 20% – 35% of the daily cal, as per the 2015 to 2020 Dietary Guidelines for Americans. Saturated fat does not allow for more than 10 percent of daily cal.

Depending on the form of fat, it may be fine, evil, or anywhere in the middle.

Trans fats, for example, rise in ammation, lower levels of "good" cholesterol, and raise levels of "bad" cholesterol. Cooked foods and baked products include them.

Saturated fats have been linked to an increased risk of heart failure. Experts, on the other hand, have differing viewpoints on this. It is prudent to consume them in moderation. Saturated fats are abundant in whole milk, red meat, coconut oil, and baked goods.

Polyunsaturated and monounsaturated fats are examples of healthy fats. These fats have been shown to lower the risk of heart failure, reduce blood pressure, and lower lipid content in the blood.

These fats are abundant in peanut oil, olive oil, sunflower oil, canola oil, safflower oil, and soybean oils.

The Intermittent fasting food list for the fats include:

- Nuts

- Avocados
- Whole eggs
- Cheese
- Chia seeds
- Dark chocolate
- Full-fat yogurt
- Extra virgin olive oil

To Promote Gut Health

Gut health is linked to physical health, according to a growing body of proof. The microbiota is a set of billions of bacteria that live in your stomach.

Gut hygiene, metabolism, and emotional health are all affected by these microbes. They may also be essential in the treatment of a variety of chronic illnesses.

As a result, you should keep an eye on those pesky bugs in the stomach, particularly if you're fasting intermittently.

The IF food list for a normal and healthy gut include:

- Fermented vegetables
- All vegetables
- Kombuch
- Tempeh
- Kimchi
- Sauerkraut
- Miso

In order to keep the gut healthy, the foods mentioned above may also aid you to lose weight by:

- Increasing the ingested fat excretion through stools.
- Reducing the fat absorption from your gut.
- Reducing the food intake.

For Hydration

The regular criteria, as per the National Academies of Medicines, Engineering, and Science, is:

For adults, 15.5 cups (3.7 l) is right.

For ladies, 11.5 cups (2.7 l) is right.

Water, as well as water-containing foods and beverages, are considered fluids.

It's important to stay hydrated during intermittent fasting for your wellbeing. Headaches, severe tiredness, and brain fog are all symptoms of dehydration. If you're still suffering from these fasting adverse effects, dehydration will cause them worse or even fatal.

The IF food list for the hydration include:

- Sparkling water
- Water
- Watermelon
- Strawberries
- Tea or Black coffee
- Peaches
- Cantaloupe

- Skim milk
- Plain yogurt
- Oranges
- Cucumber
- Lettuce
- Tomatoes
- Celery

Drinking plenty of water may also aid with weight loss. A 2016 research shows that proper hydration may aid you to lose weight by:

- Increasing fat burning.
- Decreasing the food intake or appetite.

Foods To Avoid from The IF Food List

- Trans-fat
- Processed foods
- Candy bars
- Sugar-sweetened beverages
- Alcoholic beverages
- Processed meat

Things To Do by Using Intermittent Fasting for Specific Diets

Some people claim that mixing intermittent fasting with other diets, such as the ketogenic diet or a vegetarian diet, can help them lose weight quicker. However, whether or not this is so also up for debate.

If you want to consider combining IF and the keto diet? Consider the following foods in your high-fat, low-carb intermittent fasting meal list:

For Fats (75 Percent of The Daily Calories)

- Nuts
- Avocados
- Whole eggs
- Cheese
- Chia seeds
- Dark chocolate
- Full-fat yogurt
- Extra virgin olive oil

For Protein (20 Percent of The Daily Calories)

- Seafood
- Eggs
- Dairy products, for example, yogurt, cheese, and milk
- Beans and legumes
- Seeds and nuts
- Whole grains
- Soy

For Carbs (5 Percent of The Daily Calories)

- Beetroots
- Sweet potatoes

- Oats
- Brown rice
- Quinoa

The Food List for IF Vegetarian Diet May Include:
For Protein

- Seeds and nuts
- Whole grains
- Dairy products, for example, yogurt, cheese, and milk
- Soy
- Beans and legumes

For Carbs

- Beetroots
- Sweet potatoes
- Quinoa
- Brown rice
- Oats
- Mangoes
- Bananas
- Apples
- Kidney beans
- Berries
- Pears
- Carrots
- Broccoli

- Avocado
- Almonds
- Brussels sprouts
- Chickpeas
- Chia seed

For Fats
- Nuts
- Avocados
- Dark chocolate
- Cheese

3.5 Intermittent Fasting Hacks That Are Both Basic yet Effective

There has never been any eating pattern that is as consistent over the past few years, which has benefited so many people.

It has a lot of excitement about it.

Its advantages to our wellbeing are undeniable.

It is widely used to help people lose weight. The explanation for this is simple: you miss one meal a day, which is usually breakfast.

This results in a 600-800 calorie reduction. It may be an important way to lose weight when combined with a greater degree of exercise and activities.

The benefit is that it is not a typical diet in which you would consume less in order to reduce weight.

You concentrate on not consuming for a set period and instead of having water.

This would speed up the fat-burning process in your body. Your body receives the message: There isn't any food, so I'll have to depend on my fat reserves for energy.

Plus, consuming more cal than you burn in just a small time frame is more difficult than eating all day.

Lower blood sugar levels, lower blood pressure, reduced inflammation, greater insulin response, and Autophagy are other advantages.

Autophagy is indeed an evolutionary cell-recovery process that the body initiates after 10 - 12 hours of fasting, lasting up to 16 hours.

Scientists recently discovered this influence. They believe that is one of the most important advantages of intermittent fasting that will significantly increase your life expectancy when paired with a healthier lifestyle.

Why is fasting helpful to your health?

Our stone-age forefathers did not have the same access to calories that we do today.

They were unable to shop for food at the store. They couldn't go to a McDonald's drive-in and buy burgers to XXL coke and have anything edible in about two minutes. There were moments where there was plenty to eat for days on end.

They'd go hunting, kill an animal, and feed the rest of their tribe. Hunting had been fruitful on occasion, though not always.

In the defeat, human nature had to devise a way to provide energy support to the body.

As a result, it accumulated fat deposits as buffers for times of starvation.

They were created to provide nutrition to the body when there was no food accessible.

Being a little chubby was essential to our species' existence. The human race could not have survived if stone-age men had become as muscular and strong as athletic bodybuilders. There'd have been no fat deposits to draw on at times of drought.

What is your motivation for fasting?

We would like to state right away that developing this habit may be difficult.

Many people want to give it a shot, but they're having trouble establishing a new schedule. If you wish to reap the rewards of intermittent fasting, you can excel and find it a very simple task. However, you should be certain of the WHY.

- What motivates you to do it?
- If you want to drop weight?
- Do you want to be more energized and less tired in the day?
- What drives you to do what you do?

It's better to write it down and post it somewhere you'll use it often, such as your workplace.

Changing your eating habits can be difficult, particularly if you are used to a voracious appetite. However, it is probable, and once introduced, you can find a difference.

The 16:8 fast, which involves 16 hours of not consuming and an 8-hour feeding window, is the most common. We have discovered a few tricks that may help you get through the 16-hour quick with minimal energy loss and hunger.

The human body is a survival mechanism that will go for days with no food until it is suffering from anorexia.

Intermittent fasting can be laid out in a variety of ways:

You could eat lunch at noon and dinner at 8 pm. This is the most widely used edition.

Other people do it from 7 am to 3 pm; they don't consume something until they go to bed.

The first choice is more preferable. It is all up to you.

The next five hacks are geared toward the variant that you begin eating in the afternoon. Begin slowly.

You don't have to slam your face into it straight away. There is no need to rush.

IF is not as simple as it might seem, and nothing useful comes easily.

It takes time to get used to it, much like every other habit. Allow the body to adjust to the latest feeding period for at least 20 - 30 days.

If you're a disciplined individual looking for a new task, starting 16:8 fasting right away might be a good idea. However, for the vast majority of people, it is preferable to begin slowly.

A 12-hour fast should be considered first, particularly if you're used to eating from the moment you wake up till you go to sleep. At first, the chance of feeling hunger pangs and reverting to your old habits is high.

Slowly but steadily increase your fasting time, one hour at a time, before you reach 16 hours.

When you've gone 16 hours without eating, treat yourself with either of your most delectable meals. Then stick with it for at least 3 - 4 weeks because it would be more difficult to revert to old habits.

Within a couple of days, you'll find changes in appearance, anxiety perception, peacefulness, less voracious appetite, and a few pounds lost on the scale.

- **A Cup of Black Coffee**

Coffee has the potential to be a powerful tool. It has no calories and will aid you on your IF journey if consumed without milk or sugar. Scientists have discovered that drinking premium coffee black and without any chemicals has fat-burning effects. Caffeine alerts the brain to the fact that it is complete. It is often prescribed during weight-loss diets for this purpose.

If you want to help with your intermittent fasting, drink 2 to 3 cups of coffee. The first one is in the morning, followed by the second and third in the mid-morning.

Tea may be substituted if you can't drink it without milk. It has a similar impact to coffee but without calories.

- **Ensure That You Consume Plenty of Water**

This is one of the most effective ways to stay on track with your fasting.

Drinking many cups of water before the first meal of the day causes weight to accumulate on your stomach walls, indicating saturation.

And if you're not doing intermittent fasting, you can drink a large glass of water first thing in the morning. Since not consuming for 8 hours and sweating the most out, the body is 70% water and needs hydration.

- **Foods That Are High in Protein**

Food with a large carbohydrate content will soon render you hungry again.

Since the insulin spike can drop faster if there are less proteins in a meal, voracious hunger attacks are more likely to occur.

Proteins are responsible for saturating the body, constructing the muscular system, and maintaining a healthy immune system.

When going on a 16-hour fast, try to stay away from high-carb and sugary foods as far as possible. Instead, consume a ton of protein-rich meals, which can make you feel less hungry and offer you more stamina.

- **Olive Oil**

You should never neglect its importance, and you should have the correct fats in your diet if you want to lose weight. They play an important role in hormone production and overall wellbeing.

People who don't consume many nutritious fat-rich foods, such as linseed and olive oil, seafood, nuts, and so on, are more likely to have hormone issues and are at a greater risk of developing a variety of diseases.

Olive oil is noted for having a variety of health benefits, including lowering blood sugar levels.

You can be less hungry in the morning if you consume 20 - 30ml of it. You can drizzle it over your meals, salads, or even consume it with a spoon.

Fasting has been very common in recent years, and its health benefits are vastly undervalued.

It's ironic that, for the majority of its life, the human body was accustomed to fasting all of the time. The new food sector is seeking to tell us differently in order to boost retail revenue.

Huge food companies, such as Nestle, want us to consume as much as possible every day for as long as possible.

Breakfast is the essential meal of the day, and similar phrases are used to persuade us that eating food after getting up is essential

We are not here to judge breakfast or some other meal, and we are aware that research has proven that eating a balanced and nutritious breakfast will help you start the day off right.

But it isn't the case every day.

There are occasions when a fast is essential.

Bear in mind that BREAK-Fast refers to the act of breaking one's fast.

Our stone-age forefathers didn't eat breakfast and seemed to survive very well. Since then, our digestive processes have also been unchanged. We have only evolved to an environment where food is accessible 24 hours a day, seven days a week. Regardless of if you choose to shed a few pounds or are ready to take on the task of changing routines, you should recommend trying fasting with the tips in this book.

Chapter 4: The Three Intermittent Fasting Programs

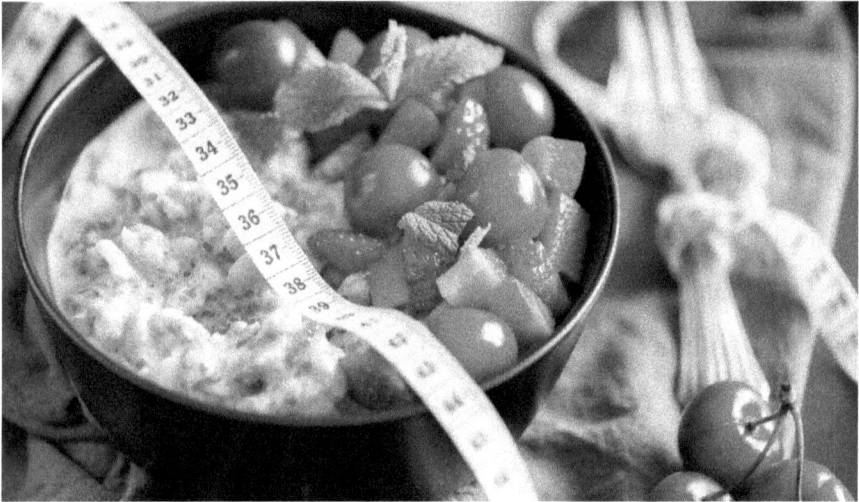

Intermittent fasting has been a common health movement in recent years. It's said to help people lose weight, boost their metabolic fitness, and maybe even live longer.

This eating trend may be approached in a variety of ways.

Any strategy has the potential to be successful, but determining which one works better for you is a personal decision.

Intermittent fasting can be done in six different forms.

4.1 The 16/8 Method

THE 16/8 METHOD

	DAY 1	DAY 2	DAY 3	DAY 4	DAY 5	DAY 6	DAY 7
Midnight 4 AM 8 AM	FAST	FAST	FAST	FAST	FAST	FAST	FAST
12 PM	First meal	First meal	First meal	First meal	First meal	First meal	First meal
4 PM	Last meal by 8pm	Last meal by 8pm	Last meal by 8pm	Last meal by 8pm	Last meal by 8pm	Last meal by 8pm	Last meal by 8pm
8 PM Midnight	FAST	FAST	FAST	FAST	FAST	FAST	FAST

The 16/8 process entails fasting for 14 to 16 hours a day and limiting your feeding window to 8 to 10 hours.

You may consume two, three, or even four meals during the feeding time.

Fitness guru Martin Berkhan popularized this form, which is also recognized as the Lean gains protocol.

It's as simple as not consuming something after dinner and missing breakfast to follow this fasting process.

If you have your last meal at 8:00 pm and don't eat again before noon the next day, you'll have fasted for 16 hours.

Women are usually advised to fast for just 14 to 15 hours since they tend to perform well with shorter fasts.

This approach can be difficult to adjust to at first for hungry people in the morning and like to consume breakfast. Many breakfast-skippers, on the other hand, feed in this manner instinctively.

You may drink coffee, water, and other low-calorie drinks during the fast, making you feel less hungry.

It's important to concentrate on consuming nutritious foods across your eating window. If you eat a lot of fast food or consume an unhealthy number of calories, this approach will not succeed.

Summary Of the 16/8 Approach:

Men are fasting for 16 hours, and women are fasting for 14–15 hours each day. You'll limit your eating to an eight to 10-hour span per day, during which you'll take in two meals.

Three or more meals are recommended.

4.2 The 5:2 Diet

THE 5:2 DIET

DAY 1	DAY 2	DAY 3	DAY 4	DAY 5	DAY 6	DAY 7
Eats normally	Women: 500 calories Men: 600 calories	Eats normally	Eats normally	Women: 500 calories Men: 600 calories	Eats normally	Eats normally

The 5:2 diet entails regularly eating five days a week and limiting your calorie consumption to 500 to 600 calories on the other two days.

Michael Mosley, a British reporter, popularized this diet, also known as the Quick Diet.

On fasting days, women should consume 500 cal, and men should consume 600 cal.

You may, for example, regularly eat every day except Thursdays and Mondays. You consume two small meals of 250 cal each for women and 300 cal each for men for those two days.

No trials evaluate the 5:2 diet itself, as opponents rightly point out, but there are loads of studies about intermittent fasting advantages.

Summary Of the 5:2 Diet Approach:

Diet consists of consuming 500 to 600 calories two days a week

The remaining five days are usually off.

4.3 Eat Stop Eat

DAY 1	DAY 2	DAY 3	DAY 4	DAY 5	DAY 6	DAY 7
Eats normally	24-hour fast	Eats normally	Eats normally	24-hour fast	Eats normally	Eats normally

Once maybe or twice a week, Eat Stop Eat requires a 24-hour fast.

Fitness specialist Brad Pilon popularized this form, which has been very common for a few years.

This leads to a perfect 24-hour fast if you fast from dinner one day to dinner the next day.

You've done a perfect 24-hour quick if you end dinner at 7:00 pm Monday and don't feed again before dinner at 7:00 pm Tuesday. The outcome is the same if you fast from lunch to lunch or breakfast to breakfast.

During the fast, liquids such as coffee, water, and other low-calorie drinks are tolerated, but solid foods are not.

You must diet normally during the feeding cycles while you're trying to lose weight. In other words, you can consume as much as you would if you weren't fasting at all.

A complete 24-hour fast can be challenging for certain individuals, which is a possible disadvantage to this approach. You don't have to go all-in right away, however. It's perfect, to begin with, 14 to 16 hours and work your way up.

Summary Of the Eat Stop Eat Approach:

An IF program with 1 or 2 24-hour fasts every week.

4.4 Alternate-Day Fasting

ALTERNATE-DAY FASTING

DAY 1	DAY 2	DAY 3	DAY 4	DAY 5	DAY 6	DAY 7
Eats normally	24-hour fast OR Eat only a few hundred calories	Eats normally	24-hour fast OR Eat only a few hundred calories	Eats normally	24-hour fast OR Eat only a few hundred calories	Eats normally

You fast every single day as you practice alternate-day fasting. This approach is available in a variety of forms. During fasting days, some of them make around 500 calories.

This technique was used in several of the test-tube trials that showed the health effects of intermittent fasting.

A complete fast any other day may seem excessive, so it is not suggested for beginners.

This approach can cause you to go to bed hungry numerous times a week, which is unpleasant and unlikely to be sustainable in the long run.

Summary Of the Alternate-Day Fasting Approach:

It makes you fast every day, either by not consuming something or only eating a couple of hundred calories a day.

4.5 The Warrior Diet

THE WARRIOR DIET

	DAY 1	DAY 2	DAY 3	DAY 4	DAY 5	DAY 6	DAY 7
Midnight							
4 AM	Eating only small amounts of vegetables and fruits	Eating only small amounts of vegetables and fruits	Eating only small amounts of vegetables and fruits	Eating only small amounts of vegetables and fruits	Eating only small amounts of vegetables and fruits	Eating only small amounts of vegetables and fruits	Eating only small amounts of vegetables and fruits
8 AM							
12 PM							
4 PM	Large meal	Large meal	Large meal	Large meal	Large meal	Large meal	Large meal
8 PM							
Midnight							

Ori Hofmekler popularized the Warrior Diet.

In this diet, you just consume vegetables and fruit at lunch and dinner.

All you have to do is fast all day and feed within a four-hour feeding time.

The Warrior Diet was among the first IF diets to be successful. This lifestyle has many of the same principles as the paleo diet — mainly whole, unprocessed ingredients.

Summary Of the Warrior Diet Approach:

The Warrior Diet recommends consuming few tiny portions of fruits and vegetables per day and then a big meal each night.

4.6 Spontaneous Meal Skipping

SPONTANEOUS MEAL SKIPPING

DAY 1	DAY 2	DAY 3	DAY 4	DAY 5	DAY 6	DAY 7
Breakfast	Skipped Meal	Breakfast	Breakfast	Breakfast	Breakfast	Breakfast
Lunch	Lunch	Lunch	Lunch	Lunch	Lunch	Lunch
Dinner	Dinner	Dinner	Dinner	Skipped Meal	Dinner	Dinner

You don't need to pursue a formal intermittent fasting regimen to enjoy any of the rewards. Also, one can choose to go a day or two without food, such as when you are busy and don't want to feed.

The idea that people ought to feed every few hours in order to avoid hitting hunger mode or losing muscle doesn't have much validity. you can go for long stretches without food without causing the body a hard time

If you aren't very hungry on the day, have a good breakfast but a light lunch and dinner. Whether you'll be out and don't have something you like to consume, have a small or no meal.

This is essentially an intermittent fast, whether you miss only one or two meals.

Be sure you consume nutritious foods on other occasions per day.

Summary Of the Spontaneous Meal Skipping Approach:

An alternative to the traditional intermittent fasting approach is to miss one or two meals when you're not hungry or do not have the opportunity.

Please Note

Though intermittent fasting may be an effective tool for weight loss, some people think it's not effective for women. Individuals who've or are predisposed to eating disorders should avoid them.

You may want to give it a shot, so choose your diet carefully. You cannot afford to consume unhealthy foods while on the times you are consuming, and expect to get healthy results.

Chapter 5: How to Develop an Appropriate Fasting Program

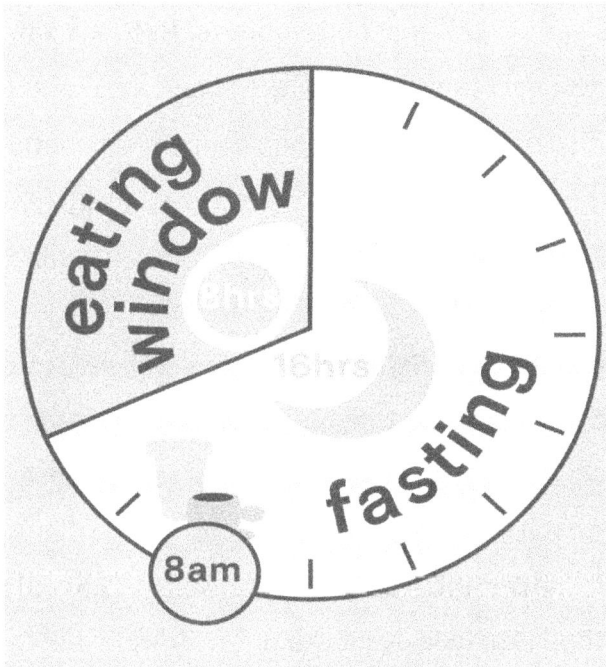

5.1 The Simplest Way to Begin Intermittent Fasting

The easiest way to get you started on Intermittent Fasting on the right foot and prevent errors is to emphasize the value of consuming clean whole foods when you're fasting.

But first, let's have a look at the different forms of fasting so you can figure out which one is right for you. That is crucial, as you are aware. Choose the strategy that you believe would give you the best results and get started. Both of the choices are viable, depending on the lifestyle and end goals. Let's get started:

- **The 16/8 Method:** Which entails fasting for 16 hours and eating well for the remaining 8. Break the fast at 12 am the next day after eating the last meal at 8 pm.

- **The 5/2 Technique:** You regularly consume five days of the week and only select meals that are 500 to 600 calories a day for the remaining two days (250 to 300 cal each meal).

- **The Stop-Eat-Stop Strategy:** You fast for 24 hrs once or twice a week in this regimen. If you're used to feeding three or four meals a day, this could be a daunting approach to adopt at first.

- **The Alternate-Day Approach:** The rule of this method is to feed every other day. It's normal to consume 500 cal on fasting days and consume whatever you want on non-fasting days.

- **The Random Meal Skipping Process:** This IF method entails skipping meals when required. You will gain from it even if it is not a regimented system.

5.2 Benefits of Intermittent Fasting

It's important to consider the impact of a fasting diet on your body in order to remain on board and achieve your goals. Knowing what to expect will help you stay motivated while you adapt to IF.

- Since you are not eating to raise blood glucose levels, Intermittent Fasting lowers insulin levels. As a result, the body draws nutrition from fat reserves.
- Improved blood supply to the brain increases neurological and emotional sharpness.
- The Energy Levels Would Rise.
- Human Growth Hormone levels rise, which has a beneficial impact on muscular mass growth and bone density.
- As aged cells die, they are fixed and substituted.
- The kidneys help to reduce blood pressure by removing extra salt and water. This further aids in the reduction of inflammation within the body.
- The amount of bad cholesterol (LDL) decreases, whereas the amount of good cholesterol (HDL) is raised.

5.3 If Mistakes and Ways to Avoid Them

- **Getting Off Quickly with Intermittent Fasting**

One of the greatest errors you can create is to start so quickly. You will set yourself up for failure if you hop into IF without first easing into it. It may be difficult to transition from consuming three normal meals or six small meals a day to consuming within a four-hour timeframe, for example.

Instead, eventually, introduce fasting. If you choose to use the 16/8 process, gradually increase the period between meals so you can function easily in 12 hours. Then, to bring the window down to 8 hours, add a few minutes per day before you get there.

- **Choose The Wrong Intermittent Fasting Plan**

You've shopped for whole foods like fish and poultry, fruits and vegetables, and nutritious sides like legumes and quinoa, and you're willing to pursue Intermittent Fasting for weight loss. The issue is that you haven't selected the IF strategy that will ensure your performance. If you go to the gym six days a week, absolutely fasting on two of those days might not be the best option for you.

Rather than jumping into a strategy without worrying about it, examine your lifestyle and choose the plan that better fits your routine and behaviors.

- **Excessive Eating in The Fasting Window**

The shortened time left to consume requires eating less calories, which is one reason individuals want to pursue Intermittent Fasting. On the other hand, some individuals may consume their usual number of calories during the fasting window. It's possible that you won't lose weight as a result of this.

Don't consume the daily calorie intake of 2000 cal in the slot. Instead, aim for a caloric intake of 1200 - 1500 cal during the time you're breaking the fast. If you fast for four, six, or eight hours, the number of meals you consume can be determined by the fasting window duration. If you find yourself in a state of starvation and need to feed, rethink the diet you want to pursue, or take a day off the IF to concentrate, then get back on track.

- **In Fasting Window, Eating the Wrong Foods**

Overeating goes hand and hand with the Intermittent Fasting error of consuming the wrong things. You would not feel good if you've a fasting time of six hours and fill it with processed, salty, or sugary foods.

Your diet's mainstay becomes lean meats, good fats, almonds, legumes, unprocessed grains, and wholesome vegetables and fruits. Also, while you're not fasting, keep some healthy food ideas in mind:

Rather than eating at a pub, cook and eat at home.

Read diet labels and learn about additives, including high fructose corn syrup and refined palm oil that isn't allowed.

Keep an eye out for hidden sugars and restrict sodium consumption.

Instead of refined ingredients, prepare whole foods.

Fiber, balanced carbohydrates and fats, and lean protein can all be present on your plate.

- **Calorie Limitation in The Fasting Window**

And, there is such a phenomenon as calorie restriction that is excessive. It's not safe to eat fewer than 1200 cal during your fasting window. Not just that, but it has the potential to slow down your metabolic rate. If you delay your metabolism so long, you'll start losing muscle mass instead of gaining it.

To stop making this error, plan your meals for the week ahead on the weekend. You'll have balanced, nutritious meals at your fingertips in no time. When it's time to eat, you can choose from various good, tasty, and calorie-balanced options.

- **Breaking Intermittent Fast Without Realizing It**

It's necessary to be conscious of secret fast breakers. Did you realize that even the flavor of sugar makes the brain release insulin? This triggers the release of insulin, essentially breaking the high. Here are some unexpected foods, supplements, and items that can stop a fast and trigger an insulin response:

1. Supplements containing pectin and maltodextrin as well as other additives
2. Sugar and fat are used in supplements such as gummy bear vitamins.
3. Using mouthwash and toothpaste with xylitol as a sweetener
4. Sugar can be used in the wrapping of pain relievers like Advil.

Breaking the fast is a common Intermittent Fasting error. When you're not feeding, clean your teeth with a baking soda and water mixture, and review the labels closely before consuming supplements and vitamins.

- **Drinking Insufficiently During Intermittent Fasting**

IF necessitates that you stay hydrated. Keep in mind that the body isn't absorbing the water that will normally be absorbed with food. As a result, if you're not patient, side effects might throw you off. If you encourage yourself to be dehydrated, you can experience nausea, muscle cramps, and extreme hunger.

Also include following in the day to prevent this error to avoid unpleasant signs including cramping and headaches:

1. water

2. 2 tbsp. apple cider vinegar and water (this might even curb your hunger)
3. a cup of black coffee
4. Green tea, black tea, herbal tea, oolong tea

- **When Intermittently Fasting, People Don't Really Exercise**

Some people assume they can't exercise during an IF time when it's the perfect circumstance. Exercising makes you burn fat that has been accumulated in your body. Additionally, when you exercise, the Human Growth Hormone levels rise, assisting in muscle growth. There are, though, certain guidelines to obey to get the most out of the workouts.

Keep the following points in mind to achieve the maximum outcomes from your efforts:

1. Time your workouts to coincide with meal times, and only consume nutritious carbohydrates and proteins within thirty minutes of finishing your workout.
2. If the workout is strenuous, make sure you feed beforehand to replenish the glycogen reserves.
3. Focus the workout on the fasting method; if you're fasting for 24 hours, don't do something strenuous every day.
4. During the swift, and particularly during the exercise, stay hydrated.

5. Pay attention to the body's signals; if you start to feel tired or lightheaded, take a rest or stop working out.

- **Becoming So Hard on Yourself While Intermittently Fasting If You Slip**

One blunder does not mean loss! You'll have days where an IF diet is especially difficult, and you do not think you'll be able to keep up. It's perfectly acceptable to take a break if necessary. Set aside a day to refocus. Stick to the balanced food plan, but indulge in surprises like an amazing protein smoothie or a plate of nutritious broccoli and beef the next day.

Don't slip into the pit of having Intermittent Fasting take over your whole life. Consider it a part of your good routine; just don't forget to take care of yourself in other ways. Enjoy a book, read, get some exercise, spend more time with your mates, and live as healthily as possible. It's just part of the process of being the strongest version of yourself.

Chapter 6: How to Exercise Safely During Intermittent Fasting

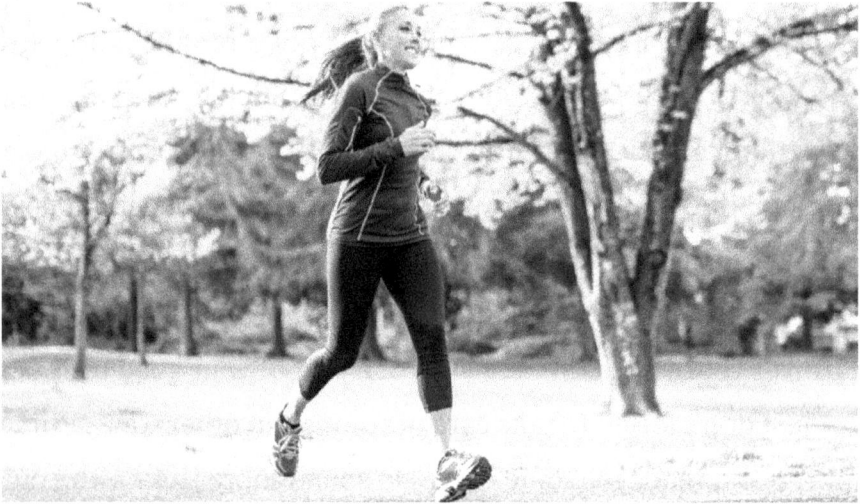

6.1 The Benefits and Risks of Exercising Whilst on A Fast

Whether you're new to intermittent fasting or fasting for some cause and want to keep working out, there are a few pros and cons to remember when deciding to exercise when fasting.

According to certain studies, exercise while fasting changes muscle biochemistry and metabolism, which are related to insulin sensitivity and blood sugar level control.

Eating and exercising right afterward, until digestion or absorption, has often been shown to be beneficial. This is especially significant for people who have type 2 diabetes or suffer from metabolic syndrome.

According to Chelsea Amengual, one advantage of fasting is that your accumulated carbs, identified as glycogen, are more definitely exhausted, meaning you will be burning more fat to fuel your exercise.

Does the prospect of burning more fat sound appealing? There is a drawback to the fasted cardio trend that you should be aware of before jumping on board.

It's likely that if you work out when fasted, the body may start breaking down muscle and use protein as food, according to Amengual. "And as well as, you're more likely to hit a wall," she continues, "which ensures you will have less stamina and won't be able to work out as much or do as well."

IF and long-term exercise isn't suitable. "The body reduces itself of calories and power, which may cause the metabolism to slow down," she continues.

Should You Exercise While Fasting?

- You would be able to burn more fat.
- If you fast for an extended period of time, your metabolism can slow down.
- You might not be able to provide the best effort during workouts.

- You can lose muscle mass or just be able to retain muscle mass rather than develop it.

6.2 Getting A Good Workout Session While Fasting

If you choose to pursue intermittent fasting while continuing to exercise, there are a few items you can do to keep your workout more successful.

- **Consider The Pacing**

When it comes to getting the workout more successful when fasting, there are three things to consider: whether you can exercise before, after, or after the fueling window.

The 16:8 protocol is a common IF form. The idea entails eating everything during an 8-hour fueling timeframe before fasting for 16 hours.

"Exercising before the window is best for someone who does well during a workout on an empty stomach, and working out during the window is good for someone who does not want to work out on an empty stomach but needs to take advantage of post-workout nutrition," he says. During is the safest choice for success and regeneration, according to Shuff.

He continues, "After the window is for those who want to work out after fueling but do not have time to do so during the feeding window."

- **Decide The Sort of Exercise You Can Perform Depending on Your Macros**

Lynda Lippin, a licensed fitness trainer, says it's essential to give attention to the macronutrients you consume the day before and after your workout.

Power exercises, for example, necessitate further carbs on the day of the exercise, while cardio/high-intensity interval workouts may be performed on a lower carb day, she describes.

- **To Develop or Sustain Strength, Eat the Right Foods During the Exercise**

According to Dr. Niket Son pal, the easiest way to combine IF and fitness is to schedule your exercises during your eating cycles so that your nutrition levels are at their highest. "It's also essential for the body to have protein after such a heavy lifting exercise to help in regeneration," he continues. Amengual recommends eating carbs and around 20 g of protein within thirty minutes of the workout following some strength exercise.

6.3 How Do You Work Out Comfortably While Fasting?

Any weight reduction or fitness program's effectiveness is determined by how safe it is to maintain over time. Keep in the safe zone if your overall aim is to shed body fat and preserve your health level when doing IF. Here are few professional suggestions to assist you in doing so.

- **Closely Follow the Mild- To High-Intensity Exercise with A Meal**

This is when the value of meal preparation falls into action. It's crucial, according to Khorana, to eat prior to a low- or high-intensity exercise. As a consequence, the body may have some glycogen supplies to draw from to power your exercise.

- **Keep Yourself Hydrated**

It's important to note that fasting does not imply dehydration, according to Sonpal. In reality, he advises drinking more water when fasting.

- **Maintain A Healthy Electrolyte Balance**

Coconut water, according to Sonpal, is a healthy, low-calorie hydration source. He claims that it replenishes electrolytes, tastes nice, and is low in cal. Stop consuming too much Gatorade or athletic beverages since they are rich in sugar.

- **Maintain A Low Level of Intensity and Duration**

Take a rest if you feel lightheaded or dizzy after pushing yourself so hard. It's important to pay attention to the body. Think of the kind of fast you'll be doing.

If you're doing a 24-hour sporadic fast, Lippin recommends doing low-intensity exercises like:

1. Jogging
2. Yoga for relaxation
3. Pilates is a gentle workout

However, since most of the 16-hour fasting window is spent in the evening, sleeping, and early in the morning if you are doing the 16:8 fast, keeping to a certain form of workout isn't as essential.

6.4 Pay Attention to The Body

When exercising during Intermittent fasting, the essential thing to remember is to listen to your body.

"If you tend to feel tired or dizzy, it's likely that you have low blood sugar level or are dehydrated," Amengual says. If that's the case, she recommends starting with a carb-electrolyte drink and then eating a well-balanced lunch.

Although exercising and IF can be beneficial to certain individuals, others might be uncomfortable exercising at all while fasting.

Before beginning any diet or fitness regimen, consult the doctor or healthcare professional.

6.5 Is It Possible to Lose Weight Faster If You Exercise with An Empty Stomach?

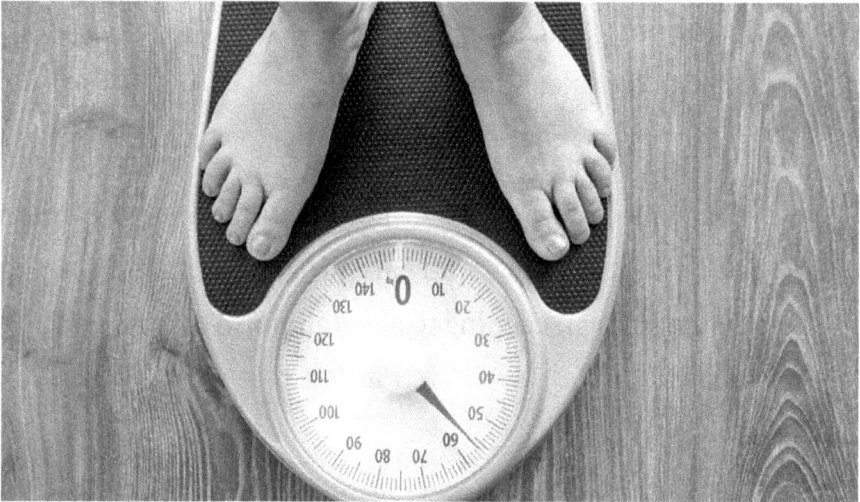

Have you ever been advised to exercise with an empty stomach? Fasted cardio, or cardio performed before or after eating, is a common subject in the health and diet community.

There are supporters and detractors, as with many wellness phenomena.

Some individuals swear it as a quick and easy way to lose weight, whilst others think it's a waste of time and effort.

Fasted cardio does not often indicate that you're pursuing an intermittent fasting schedule. It may be as easy as heading on a run first thing in the morning and then having breakfast.

The advantages and pitfalls of fasted cardio were addressed with three health and diet experts. This is what they have to suggest about it.

- **Giving It a Shot:** You might be able to burn more fat if you do any fasted cardio.

In weight loss and exercise circles, using the treadmill or upright cycle for a workout session before eating is popular. The prospect of losing more fat is often the primary motivator. So how does it work in practice?

Emmie Satrazemis, a board-licensed sports nutritionist, says, "Not getting extra calories or food on hand from either a recent meal or a pre-workout snack pushes the body to focus on stored fuel, which tends to be glycogen and stored fat."

Exercise in the morning after fasting for 8 - 12 hours through sleep, according to a reputable source, will help you burn up to 20 percent more fat. However, some studies indicate it has little effect on total fat loss.

- **Skip It:** If you're looking to gain muscle mass, consuming before a cardio exercise is necessary.

However, there is a distinction to be made between gaining muscle mass and maintaining muscle mass.

"As long as you consume enough protein and use your muscles, it shows that muscle mass is very well maintained, even in a cal deficit," Satrazemis explains.

That is because amino acids aren't as ideal as stored carbohydrates and fat while your body is searching for food. Satrazemis, on the other hand, claims that the supply of instant energy is minimal and that exercising too hard for too long when fasting can cause you to run out of energy or begin to break down more muscle.

She also claims that eating after a workout helps you regenerate these stores and heal the muscle damage that happened during your workout.

- **Giving It a Shot:** You love the way fasted cardio helps your body sound.

This explanation can seem self-evident, but it's not unusual to wonder why we do things, even though they make you happy. As a result, Satrazemis believes that the choice to pursue fasted cardio is a personal one. "Some people like to exercise on an empty stomach, whilst others do best while they eat," she explains.

- **Don't Do It:** Activities that demand a lot of strength and pace can be done with food in the stomach.

As per David Chesworth, an ACSM-licensed fitness trainer, if you intend on doing an exercise that requires high amounts of strength or pace, you can eat before doing certain exercises.

He explains why glucose is the best fuel for strength and pace operations since it is the fastest energy type. "The physiology does not usually provide the optimal tools for this form of work out in a fasted state," Chesworth adds. As a result, if you want to get quick and strong, he recommends training once you have eaten.

- **Give It a Shot:** If you're dealing with GI issues, fasted cardio can be beneficial.

If you eat a meal or maybe even a snack before performing the exercise, you can feel nauseous throughout your workout. "This is particularly valid in the morning, as well as with high fiber and high-fat foods," Satrazemis says.

If you can't afford a bigger meal or don't have at least two days to process it, you might be best served eating anything with a simple energy supply or doing exercise when fasted.

- **Don't Do It:** You have a medical problem.

You must be in outstanding shape to do cardio in a fasted condition. You should also remember health issues like low blood pressure or low blood sugar, which may induce dizziness and place you at risk for injuries, according to Satrazemis.

6.6 Tips for Performing Fasted Cardio

If you wish to attempt fasted cardio, keep the following guidelines in mind to ensure your safety:

- Do not exercise for more than 60 minutes without consuming.
- Choose exercises that are mild to low-intensity.
- Drinking water is a part of fasted cardio, so remain hydrated.
- Remember that your overall lifestyle, particularly your diet, has a greater impact on your weight loss or gain than your workouts' frequency.
- Pay attention to health and do what feels right. If you're unsure whether or not you can perform fasted cardio, seek advice from a licensed nutritionist, personal trainer, or doctor.

6.7 Types of IF That Are Best for Women

There is no such thing as a one-size-fits-all solution to dieting. This is valid with extended fasting as well.

Women can, on average, take a calmer approach to fast than men.

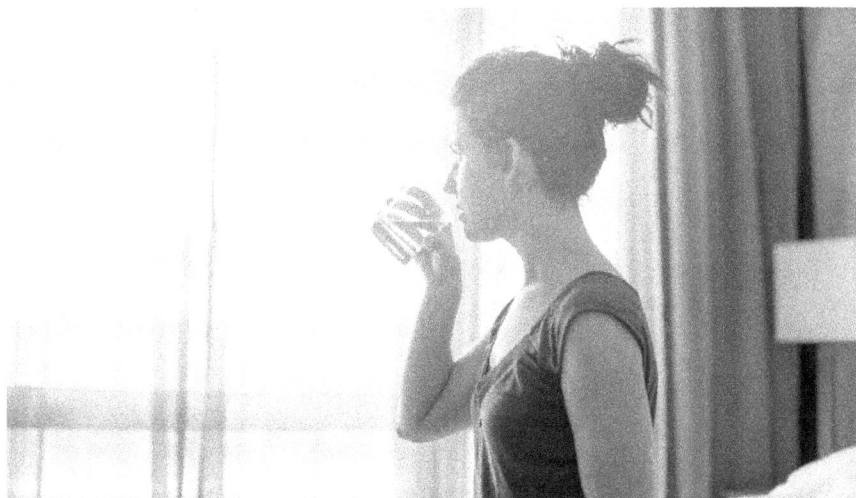

Shorter fasting times, less fasting days, and eating a limited amount of cal on fasting days are also potential choices.

Here are a few of the better intermittent fasting options for women:

- **Crescendo Method**

12–16 hours Fasting twice a week for 2 to 3 days. Fasting days should not be concurrent and should be spread out uniformly across the week (Mon, Wed and Fri).

- **The Eat-Stop-Eat Protocol (Also Known as the 24-Hour Protocol)**

Once maybe or twice a week, go on a complete 24-hour easy (max of 2 times a week for women). Begin with 14 to 16-hour fasts and work your way up.

- **5:2 Diet (Also Known as "The Quick Diet")**

Two days a week, limit cal to 25 percent of your usual diet

(approximately 500 cal) and eat regularly the other five days. Fasting days can be separated by one day.

- **Updated Alternate-Day Fasting**

Alternate days are fasting but regularly consuming on non-fasting days. On a fasting day, you are required to eat 20–25 percent of your normal calorie intake (roughly 500 calories).

- **The 16/8 Method (Also Known as the "Lean gains Approach")**

This involves fasting for sixteen hours a day and consuming all of the Cals within 8 hours. Women can begin with 14-hour fasts and work their way up to 16 hours.

It is also necessary to eat well throughout the non-fasting hours, regardless of which option you chose. You do not enjoy the same weight reduction and health effects if you consume a lot of fatty, calorie-dense items during non-fasting times.

At the end of your day, the right approach is something that you can handle and maintain over time while not causing any detrimental health effects.

Conclusion

Intermittent fasting is a form of eating that switch between fasting and eating times. It doesn't tell you the foods to consume, but rather when you can eat them.

In this way, it's more aptly defined as an eating style rather than a diet in common sense. Regular fasting for 24 hours or 16-hour fasts twice a week are two popular intermittent fasting practices.

Intermittent fasting is one of the most influential health and wellness phenomena in the world right now. People are using it to lose weight, strengthen their wellbeing, and ease their lives. Intermittent fasting's health advantages are due to improvements in hormone levels, cell structure, and gene expression.

Human growth hormone levels increase while insulin levels decline as you fast. Cells of the body also alter gene expression and activate critical cellular repair processes. Intermittent fasting helps to navigate the steep roller coaster of menopause. If you're feeling exhaustion, insulin tolerance, or weight gain as a consequence of menopause, you might want to give it a shot.

Intermittent fasting functions on all sides of the calorie calculation. It raises the metabolic rate (calories expended), thereby decreasing the food amount you consume (reduces calories).

In recent decades, type 2 diabetes has become extremely widespread. Elevated blood sugar levels in the sense of insulin resistance are the most prominent characteristic.

Something that lowers insulin tolerance and protects against type 2 diabetes may help lower blood sugar levels. Intermittent fasting has been found to have significant benefits for insulin tolerance and to result in a significant decrease in blood sugar levels. Intermittent fasting has been shown to lower fasting blood sugar by 3 to 6 percent and fasting insulin by 20 to 31 percent in human trials.

Intermittent fasting has several health advantages for both the body and mind. It will help you lose weight while still lowering the chances of developing type 2 diabetes, cardiac failure, and cancer. It can even assist you in living a longer life.